HEALTHY KIDNEY COOKBOOK

A COMPLETE COOKBOOK WITH HEALTHY KIDNEY GUIDELINES, TIPS AND STRATEGIES FOR A GOOD MEAL PREP. DETAILED MONTHLY PLAN FOR THE KIDNEY DIET.

Table of Contents

Introduction 1

Chapter 1: Nutrition for a Healthy Kidney 5

    Food Choices to Follow 8

    Tips and Strategies to Get Better 12

    Foods to Avoid 17

    Foods that Help Improve the Organ 18

Chapter 2: Weekly Plan on How to Diet 24

    1 Week Diet Plan 24

    Shopping List 26

    Understand Your Nutrient Needs 29

Chapter 3: Shake and Drinks Recipes 35

    Blackberry Sage Water 35

    Berry Milk Smoothie 37

    Apple-Cinnamon Water 38

    Caramel Latte 39

    Strawberry Smoothie 40

    Watermelon Mint Drink 41

    Beet Carrot Juice 42

    Cinnamon Egg Smoothie 43

    Pineapple Sorbet Smoothie 44

    Vanilla Fruit Smoothie 45

    Protein Berry Smoothie 46

    Protein Peach Smoothie 48

    Cranberry Cucumber Smoothie 49

    Raspberry Smoothie 50

Citrus Pineapple Shake 51

Pineapple Smoothie 52

Hazelnut Coffee 53

Lemon Piña Colada 54

Blueberry Apple Blast 56

Allspice Cider 57

Chapter 4: Seafood Recipes 58

Shrimp Paella 58

Salmon & Pesto Salad 60

Baked Fennel & Garlic Sea Bass 62

Lemon, Garlic & Cilantro Tuna and Rice 63

Salmon and Sweet Potato Chowder 64

Sesame Salmon Fillets 66

Peppered Balsamic Cod 67

Seafood Gumbo 68

Salmon Chowder with Sweet Potatoes and Corn 70

Mediterranean Fish Stew 72

Tuna and Red Pepper Stew 73

Sweet and Sour Shrimp 74

Salmon with Caramelized Onions 76

Slow Cooker Shrimp in Tomato Sauce 77

Fisherman's Stew 78

Fish Chowder 79

Shrimp Creole 80

Baked Fish 81

Creamy Tuna 82

Savory Salmon Dip 83

Chapter 5: Poultry Recipes 84

Lemon & Herb Chicken Wraps 84

Carrot & Ginger Chicken Noodles 86
Rosemary and Lemon Chicken with Eggplant 87
Parsley and Turkey Cabbage Wraps 88
Turkey and Couscous Stuffed Bell Peppers 89
Zesty Caribbean Chicken 90
Cajun Chicken and Shrimp Fiesta 92
Homemade Turkey Burgers 94
Spicy Chicken Fajitas 96
Ginger and Scallion Chicken Stir Fry 98
Deep South Chicken Stew 99
Chicken with Spiced Red Cabbage and Cranberry Sauce 100
Aromatic Chicken and Eggplant Curry 102
Italian Chicken 104
Orange & Ginger Chicken Noodles 105
Lebanese Chicken Kebabs and Red Onion Salsa 107
Mediterranean Chicken and Zucchini Pasta 109
Walnut and Basil Chicken Delight 111
Chinese Chicken 112
Chicken and Mushroom Quesadillas 114

Chapter 6: Meat Recipes 116

Spiced Lamb Burgers 116
Pork Loins with Leeks 117
Chinese Beef Wraps 118
Grilled Skirt Steak 119
Spicy Lamb Curry 120
Lamb with Prunes 122
Roast Beef 124
Beef Brochettes 125
Country Fried Steak 126
Beef Pot Roast 127

Homemade Burgers 128
Slow-cooked Beef Brisket 130
Apricot and Lamb Tagine 132
Lemongrass and Coconut Beef Curry 134
Chili Crispy Beef Noodles 136
Harissa Lamb Burgers with Yogurt and Cumin Dip 138
Mighty Meatloaf 139
Pulled Pork and Apple Buns 141
Mustard and Leek Pork Tenderloin 143
Malaysian Style Lamb Curry 144

Chapter 7: Soup and Stew Recipes 145

Yucatan Soup 145
Zesty Taco Soup 147
Southwestern Posole 149
Spring Vegetable Soup 150
Seafood Corn Chowder 151
Beef Sage Soup 153
Cabbage Borscht 155
Ground Beef Soup 157
Shrimp and Crab Gumbo 158
Tangy Turkey Soup 160
Low Sodium Chicken Broth 162
Low Sodium Beef Broth 163
Creamy Potato Soup 164
Creamy Cauliflower & Butternut Squash Soup 166
Crock Pot Turkey & Sweet Potato Chipotle Chili 167
Beef &Barley Stew 168
Healthy Crockpot White Chicken Chili 169
Green Chili Stew 170
Turkey, Wild Rice, and Mushroom Soup 171

Veggie Soup 173

Chapter 8: Vegetable Recipes 174

Thai Tofu Broth 174
Delicious Vegetarian Lasagne 176
Chili Tofu Noodles 178
Curried Cauliflower 179
Chinese Tempeh Stir Fry 180
Parsley Root Veg Stew 181
Mixed Pepper Paella 183
Cauliflower Rice & Runny Eggs 184
Minted Zucchini Noodles 186
Chili Tempeh & Scallions 187
Cucumber-Carrot Salad 188
Crunchy Couscous Salad 189
Carrot and Jicama Salad 190
Green Beans with Bacon 191
Coconut & Pecan Sweet Potatoes 193
Veggie Bolognese 194
Bombay Potatoes 195
Potato & Broccoli Gratin 196
Summer Squash with Bell Pepper and Pineapple 197
Slow Cooker Eggplant Lasagna 198

Chapter 9: Egg and Animal Product Recipes 199

Mixed Pepper Mushroom Omelet 199
Chicken Egg Rolls 201
Mushroom Omelet 203
Onion Cheese Omelet 205
Eggs with Green Chilies 206
Pepperoni Omelet 207

Scrambled Turkey Eggs 208

Angel Eggs 210

Denver Omelets 211

Scrambled Eggs and Pesto 212

Chapter 10: Dessert Recipes 213

Lemon Mousse 213

Jalapeno Crisp 214

Raspberry Popsicle 215

Easy Fudge 216

Blueberry Muffins 217

The Coconut Loaf 219

Chocolate Parfait 220

Cauliflower Bagel 221

Almond Crackers 222

Cashew and Almond Butter 223

Nut and Chia Mix 224

Hearty Cucumber Bites 225

Pop Corn Bites 226

Hearty Almond Bread 227

Medjool Balls 228

Blueberry Pudding 229

Chia Seed Pumpkin Pudding 230

Parsley Souffle 231

Mug Cake Popper 232

Cinnamon Rice Pudding 233

Almond Butter Cookies 235

Conclusion 236

Introduction

The kidneys, two bean-shaped organs that are in the bottom of the ribs cage, and are often disregarded by people around the world. Not knowing of its importance and how it helps the body throughout our daily lives. The kidneys are the ones that deliberately helps us by filtering out all the toxic materials that enter our bodies. These waste materials go through the kidney like a slotted dish, managing minerals within the body and incorporating Vitamins A and D and in the process, produces urine. Simply put, without our kidneys, we can't survive. These organs keep our blood clean and our bodies hydrated.

Sadly, more than thirty million Americans have chronic kidney disease. This disease, if left untreated, leads to kidney failure. This is why Dr. Robert Porter and Dr. Elizabeth Torres are bringing you the Kidney Disease Diet so that you can learn to treat and manage kidney disease, prevent kidney failure, and live a longer and healthier life.

You can learn all about the function of the kidneys, the effects of the disease, how inflammation impacts your body for better and worse, mineral overload, the importance of protein, and more from Dr. Porter. Along with this vital information, you can learn delicious and tasty recipes for the kidney disease diet from Dr. Torres. By utilizing the information and recipes from the pages of this cookbook, you will find yourself on the path toward success.

Not only will you be able to treat your chronic kidney disease or CKD, but you will also be able to treat the conditions that commonly cause and worsen the disease, such as diabetes and high blood pressure.

What is Kidney Disease?

Before we tackle some on the deeper topics, first I know you are probably here cause you are worried about your kidney and probably has some kidney issues. So what actually qualifies as a kidney disease? Chronic kidney diseases (known as Chronic Renal Failure/Chronic Kidney Failure) is actually a much more widespread disease than most people realize.

Due to a lack of knowledge, most people fail to interpret the symptoms of renal diseases early on, and when they do, it's often too late.

Therefore, you must stay aware of the core symptoms of chronic kidney disease (CKD) as it will help you to understand if you are affected, and you can start to get proper treatment as soon as possible.

Some of the signs that you should look out for include:

- If you are having trouble concentrating or always experience fatigue, it might be because your kidneys are weak and can't filter out the impurities and toxins.

- If you are always having trouble sleeping, you might have toxins in your blood, which are causing the problem. In fact, Sleep Apnea is a very common symptom amongst individuals with chronic kidney disease.
- Healthy kidneys help to make red blood cells and remove toxins and wastes from your body while keeping your skin healthy. If you notice that you have dry and itchy skin, it might be a sign to have your kidneys checked.
- If you have the urge to urinate excessively, especially at night, your kidneys might be damaged.
- If you ever notice blood in your urine, it's an immediate sign that your kidneys are damaged. However, you should be aware that urine in the blood can also be caused by kidney stones, tumors or infections, so make sure to have your body checked as soon as possible.
- If you have difficulty urinating, it should also be considered as a sign.
- Constant lack of appetite might be a symptom of kidney disease.
- Kidney disease can lead to temperature imbalance in your body and constantly make you feel cold even in warm temperatures.

Keep in mind that these are not the only signs; there are lots of more pointers that you should keep an eye out. But regardless, if you experience any of the symptoms above for a recurring period of time, make sure to have yourself checked immediately.

What Causes Kidney Disease?

It's rather difficult to pinpoint exact actions that might cause kidney disease. Since the physiology and immunity differ from person to person, the causalities vary as well. But some of the general ones are as follows:

- People of specific ethnicity and races are more prone to have CKD, such as American Indians, Hispanics, African Americans.
- Obesity greatly increases the chance of suffering from CKD.
- Regular smoking increases the chance of CKD.
- CKD can come from natural aging.
- Having diabetes for a long time might cause CKD, as high blood sugar can damage the blood vessels in your kidneys. Almost one out of three people with diabetes are often diagnosed with CKD.
- A history of high blood pressure is one of the most common causes of kidney disease.
- If you have a history of CKD running through your family, there's a possibility that you might be affected, as well.

Chapter 1: Nutrition for a Healthy Kidney

Many people go through their lives, knowing very little about their kidneys. All they know are that they are two medium-sized organs (about the size of an orange) that are shaped similarly to a bean. You may even know that the kidneys are located on each side of your spine, directly below your rib cage. However, this is not enough information about these vital organs. After all, if you don't care for your kidneys, they can become diseased, leading to major health problems.

Their duties, they will filter an average of four liquid ounces of blood every sixty seconds. While filtering this blood, the kidneys remove extra water which will be made into urine and any waste within the blood. After the water removes the water from the blood, it directs it to the bladder to become urine. This water is transported through the ureters, which are two thin tubes made out of muscle, located on each side of the bladder. This means that your kidneys, along with your bladder and ureters, are all a part of your urinary tract.

Many people mistakenly believe the kidneys act as sponges, which is far from the truth. The kidneys do not absorb and hold onto waste and harmful compounds. Instead, the kidneys filter out these toxins so that they can be completely removed from the body. They do this with a complex system that consists of millions of nephrons, which are microscopic filters. Nephrons are comprised of two components, which are the glomerulus and the tubule. In order to cleanse the blood, the glomerulus strains it of the larger molecules from fluid and waste. After these pass through the glomerulus, they head to the tubule. As the blood travels through the tubule component of the nephrons, smaller molecules of waste are collected. Not only that, but the tubule also collects any minerals found within the blood and then transfers them back into the bloodstream. But, how are these toxins removed from the kidneys and the body so that they don't stay stuck within your organs? When the kidneys filter water from your bloodstream, it combines the water with the filtered waste and toxins, therefore allowing them to be carried to the bladder before being expelled from the body.

Some of the waste that the kidneys remove from your blood is excess acid, which is produced in your blood in order to maintain healthy levels of minerals and water. This acid affects the levels of many minerals, such as potassium, sodium, calcium, and phosphorus. When these minerals are out of balance, your body will be unable to function properly. As these minerals are electrolytes, they affect the maintenance and control of your muscles, nerves, tissues, and balance. Without the proper balance of these electrolytes, you can be in a rather dangerous situation.

Athletes are frequently aware of the importance of maintaining balanced electrolytes, as your body will naturally become depleted of these minerals as you sweat. This is the reason that sports drinks are popular. These drinks contain all the electrolytes the human body requires, allowing people to refuel on both water and minerals simultaneously. However, if you consume too many sports drinks or electrolytes in other forms, you will overload your blood and kidneys. It is important to contain a balance of electrolytes with neither too few or too many.

Along with filtering out water, maintaining electrolyte levels, and removing excess acid, your kidney provides other functions. This includes the production of red blood cells, blood pressure maintenance, hydration regulation, hormone production, vitamin D production for bone health.

Food Choices to Follow

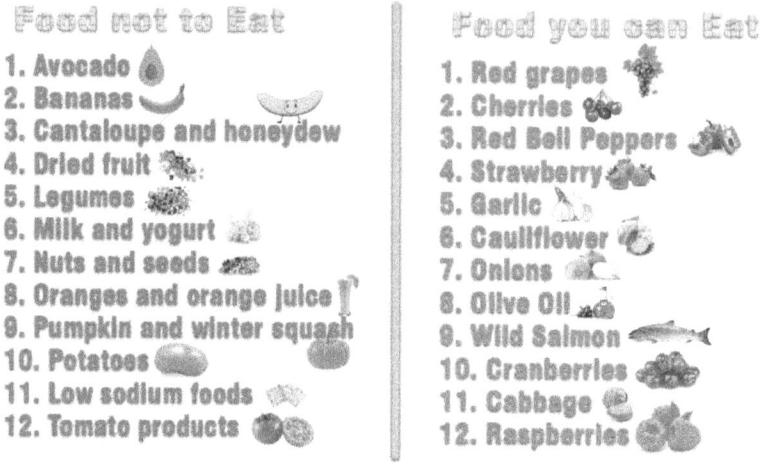

This will cover the choices you can make to ensure a healthy diet and the best treatment for your kidneys. Advice and guidance will differ according to what stage of the disease you're in, however, the principles remain similar throughout. Check with your doctor or nutritionist to ensure your diet plans are the best for you. Healthy food types and recommendations are outlined as well as food types and groups to consider avoiding or cutting down.

Carbohydrates and Fiber:

Although carbohydrates may be difficult to process at later stages of kidney disease, they provide a vital source of energy that can combat the feelings of lethargy. As a low protein diet is recommended, carbohydrates can also help to replace calories. Some carbohydrates are also sources of fiber. It is recommended that you eat at least 25 grams of fiber per day, even when suffering from stage 5 kidney disease and undergoing dialysis. You may become frustrated when trying to count your fiber levels as many high fibrous foods are also high in potassium, phosphorous and fluid (all of which are restricted).

Fats:

Fats often get a bad reputation as we don't often distinguish between healthy and unhealthy fats. Polyunsaturated and monounsaturated fats are healthy when consumed in moderation, whereas transfats and saturated fats should be avoided.

If you need to consume extra calories because of weight loss, these 'good' types of fat are great as part of a balanced diet. Too much fat, particularly transfats, can lead to a rapid increase in cholesterol, worsening symptoms experienced and also increasing your risk of heart disease. This is in turn linked to diabetes and high blood pressure, so it is always advised that you consume healthy fats in moderation and steer clear of the unhealthy fats altogether if possible. Oily fishes like tuna, salmon, and mackerel are excellent sources of these good fats. Choose oils for cooking and dressing such as coconut oil, canola oil, and olive oil, instead of sesame and vegetable oils.

Protein:

Although bodybuilders usually come to mind when we think of protein, it is actually an essential component of our diets and vital for repairing tissues, keeping infections at bay, and of course building muscle, even in the most exercise-phobic of us! If you have chronic kidney disease in the first few stages, it is still usually advised to consume protein for up to 15% of your daily diet, with carbohydrates and fats making up 85%. This is the same amount recommended for an average adult's daily intake. At stage 4 this recommendation usually decreases to only 10% protein. During stage 5, and if you are on dialysis, the dialysis will filter out the waste toxins from your body as well as protein, therefore it is crucial for you to include protein as part of your diet. Please note that you must follow your doctor's advice on how much protein you should be consuming at each stage, as it depends on various factors such as your height, weight and which stage of the disease you have. Always consult a professional for individual guidance before making any changes to your diet.

Phosphorus and Calcium:

Phosphates are salt compounds which include salt as well as other minerals; they work, as does calcium, to strengthen and keep our bones healthy. Extra phosphorous in the blood is usually removed by our kidneys, but kidney disease will prevent this process from functioning as it should. Unfortunately, it's not as simple as just removing all phosphates from your diet as they are pretty much in most foods, but we can look out for those high in phosphorous. You should typically stay away from processed foods as these often contain additives. Too much phosphorus can also lead to a calcium deficit which can, in turn, lead to the extreme bouts of itchiness that many chronic kidney disease sufferers report. If low calcium levels persist this can lead to further pain, a general weakening of the bones, and even bone disease. Your doctor may recommend taking a calcium supplement if your phosphorus levels remain too high. After this, medicines known as phosphorous binders may be required but always consult a professional.

Fluids:

As the kidneys start to decrease in functionality, waste toxins and excess liquids are not removed from the body as they should be. This may lead to your doctor recommending you limit the liquids you consume. Foods with high liquid content also need to be considered as well as the drinks you consume, for instance, fruits such as apples and pears, milk, soups, ice creams etc. This is more likely during the later stages of kidney disease and you should consult a professional for specific advice.

Potassium:

A mineral that plays an essential role in keeping your heart healthy as well as regulating water levels in the body. Again, this is another mineral that is usually removed when in excess through the kidney filtration system. Too much of one particular mineral is problematic as the kidneys just cannot remove it in the way they can when they are completely healthy. That being said, extremely low levels of potassium are also harmful and kidney disease sufferers may experience either extreme. This is unique to you so will need to be monitored by a professional. Potassium is commonly found in many fruits and vegetables - stick with watermelon, tangerines, pineapple, berries, apples, cherries, pears, grapes, and peaches as low potassium fruits.

Iron:

Anyone whose chronic kidney disease has resulted in anemia will need extra iron in their diet. Options that are high in iron include iron-fortified cereals, kidney beans, lima beans, chicken, pork, beef, and liver. As some iron-rich sources may conflict with other dietary considerations such as protein, ensure you find out from your doctor which sources of iron you can have.

Tips and Strategies to Get Better

Learning that you are suffering from kidney failure might be a difficult thing to cope with. No matter how long you have been preparing for the inevitable, this is something that will come as a shock to you.

But, as mentioned earlier, just because you have started dialysis, doesn't mean that everything that you hold dear has to come to an end!

It might be a little bit difficult at first to get yourself oriented to a new routine, but once you get into the groove, you'll start feeling much better.

Your nurses, loved ones, doctors, and co-workers will all be there to support you.

To make things easier, though, let me break down the individual types of problems that you might face and how you can deal with them.

Stress during Kidney Failure

When you are suffering from kidney failure, it's normal to be stressed out all the time. This might lead you to skip meals or even forgetting your medication, which might affect your health even more.

But you need to understand that life is full of hurdles and setbacks, and you really can't let them hold you back.

In that light, here are six tips to help you keep your stress under control:

- Make sure to take some time to just relax and unwind. Try to practice deep breathing, visualization, meditation or even muscle relaxation. All of these will help you to stay calm and keep your body healthy.

- Make sure to involve yourself in regular exercise. Take a hike, ride a bicycle or just simply take a jog. They all help. And if those aren't your thing, then you can always go for something more soothing, like tai chi or yoga.
- When you are feeling too stressed, try to call up a friend or a beloved family member and talk to them. And if that's not helping, you can always take help from a psychiatrist/counselor.
- Try to accept the things that are not under your control, and you can't change. Trying to enforce a change on something that is not within your reach will only make things worse for you. Better advice is to look for better ways of handling the situation instead of trying to change it.
- Don't put too much pressure on yourself, try to be good to yourself and don't expect much. You are a human being, after all, right? You can make mistakes, so accept that. Just try your best.
- And lastly, always try to maintain a positive attitude. Even when things go completely wrong, try to see the good instead of the bad and focus on that. Try to find things in all phases of your life that make you happy and that you appreciate, such as your friends, work, health and family, for example. You have no idea how much help a simple change of perspective can bring.

And on the topic of working out.

Exercise

Apart from the special diet, such as the Renal Diet, physical activity is another way through which you can improve the quality of your life.

This might be a little bit tough to do if you are alone, but it is very much possible. However, you should keep in mind that working out alone won't help you; you must work out and follow a well-balanced, healthy diet.

Both of these combined will go to great lengths to help you lose weight and control your disease.

In fact, a study has shown that people who try to complete 10,1000 steps per day and work out for about 2½ hours every week, while cutting down 500-800 calories per day and following a proper diet routine, have a 50% chance of reducing blood sugar to normal levels, which will further help you to stay healthy.

Common forms of exercise include:

- Stair climbing
- Tai Chi
- Stretching
- Yoga
- Cycling
- Walking

- Swimming

And so on.

To perform these normal workouts, you don't have to join a gym or even buy any sort of expensive equipment! You can simply take a walk around your streets, do yoga at home, and so on.

Just make sure to consult with your doctor to find out which exercise is suitable for you and adjust them to your dialysis routine.

Anxiety and Depression

These two are possibly the most prominent issues that you are going to face. A feeling of depression might last for a long period of time if left unattended. Anxiety might come at the same time, but it won't last for long.

Either way, mood swings will occur that will suddenly make you sad.

However, you should know that it is completely normal to feel anxious or sad when you're going through such a huge change in life. This is even more prominent if you start taking dialysis, as it will require you to completely change your daily routine and follow a different type of diet.

During this adjusting phase, you'll feel many emotions, such as anger, fear, sadness, etc.

To summarize:

The symptoms of depression are:

- Loss of interest
- Loss of any appetite
- Sleeping problems

On the other hand, symptoms of anxiety are:

- Constant sweating
- Quick breathing
- Inconsistent heartbeat
- Constant troubling thoughts

Regardless, the main thing to know is that you are not alone in this fight. Thousands of people have and are going through the same experience. Many people often feel left alone and lose the will to fight, but it doesn't have to be the same for you.

Help is always available! Try sharing with your family members, join support groups, talk to a social worker, etc.

It doesn't matter what your situation is; if you just reach out to the right person, then you will always find the help and support that you need.

Foods to Avoid

When it comes to the renal diet and keeping your kidneys healthy, the most important thing to keep in mind is to avoid foods that are high in:

- Potassium
- Phosphorus
- Sodium

That being said, the following food groups are strictly prohibited during a renal diet:

- Vitamin and mineral supplements
- Cheese
- Cream soup
- Dried beans/peas
- Ice cream
- Milk/coconut milk
- Nuts, low salt snack foods
- Peanut butter
- Nut butter
- Nutella

Foods that Help Improve the Organ

But don't be alarmed! There is still a bucket load of amazing ingredients that you can use to create awesome meals. These include:

Meat and Meat Substitutes

- Beef
- Chicken
- Fish
- Lamb

- Tuna
- Turkey
- Veal
- Pork Chops
- Tofu

Vegetables

- Beets
- Arugula
- Celery
- Chiles
- Carrots
- Asparagus
- Bean sprouts
- Chives
- Coleslaw
- Corn
- Cucumber
- Eggplants
- Endive
- Ginger root
- Green beans
- Lettuce
- Onions
- Parsley
- Radishes

- Spaghetti squash
- Turnips
- Vegetable, mixed
- Water chestnuts

Fruits

- Apricots
- Grapefruit
- Lime
- Pears
- Tangerines
- Apples
- Blackberries
- Peaches
- Pineapple
- Watermelon
- Cherries
- Figs
- Grapes
- Peach Nectar
- Raspberries
- Plums
- Apricot nectar
- Cranberries
- Fruit cocktail
- Lemon

- Pear nectar
- Strawberries

Bread and Cereals

- Corn Chex
- English muffins
- Melba toast
- Pretzels, unsalted
- Couscous
- Grits
- Noodles
- Rice/brown/white
- Kellogg's Cornflakes
- Crackers, unsalted
- Oyster crackers
- Spaghetti
- Cheerios
- Dinner rolls
- Pita Bread
- Tortillas

Fats

- Butter
- Canola oil
- Mayonnaise
- Cream cheese

- Margarine
- Miracle Whip
- Nondairy creamer
- Olive oil

Sweets

- Animal crackers
- Angel Food cake
- Candy corn
- Chewing um
- Cotton candy
- Crispy rice treats
- Graham crackers
- Gumdrops
- Gummy Bears
- Hard candy
- Hot tamales candy
- Jell-O
- Jellybeans
- Jolly Rancher
- Lemon cake
- Lifesavers
- Marshmallows
- Newtons
- Pie
- Poundcake

- Rice cakes
- Vanilla wafers

Dairy and Dairy Alternatives

- Almond milk
- Coffee-Mate
- Mocha mix
- Rice Dream
- Rich's Coffee Rich

Others

- Jelly
- Maple syrup
- Sugar, brown/white
- Honey
- Jam
- Sugar, powdered
- Corn syrup

Chapter 2: Weekly Plan on How to Diet

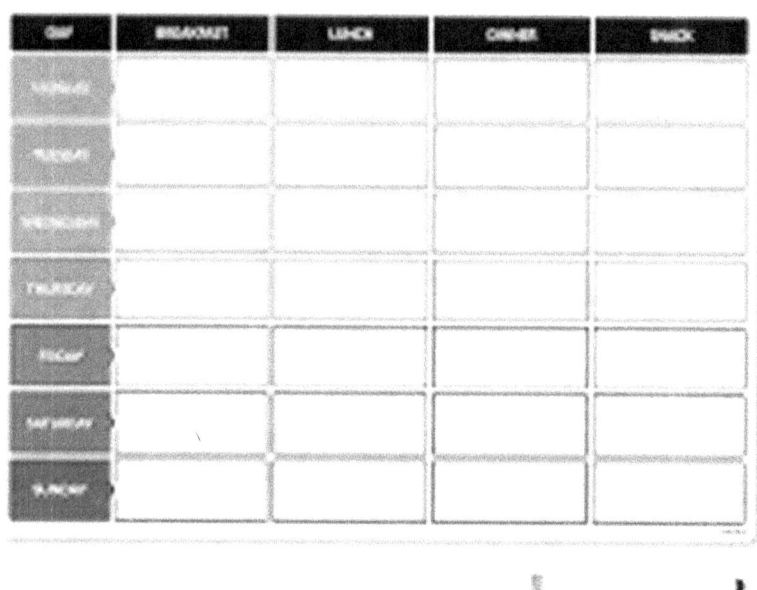

1 Week Diet Plan

Monday

Breakfast: Mixed Pepper Mushroom Omelet

Lunch: Bombay Potatoes

Dinner: Pork Loins with Leeks

Snack/Dessert: Caramel Latte

Tuesday

Breakfast: Angel Eggs

Lunch: Parsley Root Veg Stew

Dinner: Fish Chowder

Snack/Dessert: Vanilla Fruit Smoothie

Wednesday

Breakfast: Denver Omelets

Lunch: Zesty Caribbean Chicken

Dinner: Peppered Balsamic Cod

Snack/Dessert: Blueberry Apple Blast

Thursday

Breakfast: Mushroom Omelet

Lunch: Italian Chicken

Dinner: Baked Fish

Snack/Dessert: Citrus Pineapple Shake

Friday

Breakfast: Thai Tofu Broth

Lunch: Spiced Lamb Burgers

Dinner: Shrimp Paella

Snack/Dessert: Easy Fudge

Saturday

Breakfast: Slow Cooker Eggplant Lasagna

Lunch: Mighty Meatloaf

Dinner: Beef Brochettes

Snack/Dessert: Blueberry Pudding

Sunday

Breakfast: Scrambled Eggs and Pesto

Lunch: Malaysian Style Lamb Curry

Dinner: Pulled Pork and Apple Buns

Snack/Dessert: Mug Cake Popper

Shopping List

Spices and Herbs

- Oregano
- Thyme
- Onion powder
- Garlic powder
- Paprika
- Cayenne pepper
- Black pepper
- Chili powder
- Cumin
- Basil
- Rosemary

Vegetables

- Onions
- Garlic
- Carrots
- Celery
- Bell peppers
- Green beans
- Wild rice
- Beets
- Cucumbers
- Peas

Fruits

- Apples
- Pineapples
- Blueberries
- Strawberries
- Raspberries
- Cranberries
- Bananas

Meat and poultry

- Pork chops
- Beef briskets
- Chicken legs
- Chicken breasts
- Turkey breasts
- Oysters

Dairy

- Eggs
- Yogurt
- Cheese
- Low-fat milk
- Rice milk

Miscellaneous

- Chia seeds
- Farfel
- Flour
- Sesame seeds (black and white)
- Sesame oil
- Olive oil
- Cherry pie filling
- Pie crusts
- Butter
- Sweet sauce
- Hot sauce
- Splenda
- Oyster crackers
- Tortilla
- Low sodium bouillon cubes

Bad eating habits can have adverse effects on your health. If you want to avoid kidney diseases, you must manage a balanced diet and stay at a healthy weight. Your diet is supposed to contain low levels of fat and salt to control blood pressure. A diabetic person must control his/her blood sugar by choosing the right food and beverages. Control diabetes and high blood pressure to prevent the worse condition of kidney disease. Only a kidney-friendly diet can help you in the protection of kidneys from more damage. By choosing a kidney-friendly diet, you can limit particular foods to avoid the build-up of minerals in your body.

Understand Your Nutrient Needs

When following a renal diet, certain nutrients are very important as they can actually make worse or improve chronic kidney disorder. Some of the vital ones include:

Potassium

Potassium is a naturally occurring mineral found in nearly all foods, in varying amounts. Our bodies need an amount of potassium to help with muscle activity as well as electrolyte balance and regulation of blood pressure. However, if potassium is in excess within the system and the kidneys can't expel it (due to renal disease), fluid retention and muscle spasms can occur.

Phosphorus.

Phosphorus is a trace mineral found in a wide range of foods and especially dairy, meat, and eggs. It acts synergistic-ally with calcium as well as Vitamin D to promote bone health. However, when there is damage in the kidneys, excess amounts of the mineral cannot be taken out and this can cause bone weakness.

Calories

When being on a renal diet, it is important to give yourself the right amount of calories to fuel your system. The exact amount of calories you should consume daily depends on your age, gender, general health status and stage of renal disease. In most cases though, there are no strict limitations in the calorie intake, as long as you take them from proper sources that are low in sodium, potassium, and phosphorus. In general, doctors recommend a daily limit between 1800-2100 calories per day to keep weight within the normal range.

Protein

Protein is an essential nutrient that our systems need to develop and generate new connective tissue e.g. muscles, even during injuries. Protein also helps stop bleeding and supports the immune system fight infections. A healthy adult with no kidney disease would normally need 40-65 grams of protein per day.

However, in renal diet, protein consumption is a tricky subject as too much or too little can cause problems. Protein, when being metabolized by our systems also creates waste which is typically processed by the kidneys. But when kidneys are damaged or under performing, as in the case of kidney disease that waste will stay in the system. This is why patients in more advanced CKD stages are advised to limit their protein consumption as well.

Fats

Fats and particularly good fats are needed by our systems as a fuel source and for other metabolic cell functions. A diet rich in bad and trans or saturated fats though can greatly raise the odds of developing heart problems, which often occur with the renal disease. This is why most physicians advise their renal patients to follow a diet that contains a decent amount of good fats and a very low amount of trans (processed) or saturated fat.

Sodium

Sodium is an essential mineral that our bodies need to regulate fluid and electrolyte balance. It also plays a role in normal cell division in the muscles and nervous system. However, in kidney disease, sodium can quickly spike at higher than normal levels and the kidneys will be unable to expel it causing fluid accumulation as a side-effect. Those who also suffer from heart problems as well should limit its consumption as it may raise blood pressure.

Carbohydrates

Carbs act as a major and quick fuel source for the body's cells. When we consume carbs, our systems turn them into glucose and then into energy for "feeding" our body cells. Carbs are generally not restricted in the renal diet but some types of carbs contain dietary fiber as well, which helps regulate normal colon function and protect blood vessels from damage.

Dietary Fiber

Fiber is an important element in our system that cannot be properly digested but plays a key role in the regulation of our bowel movements and blood cell protection. The fiber in the renal diet is generally encouraged as it helps loosen up the stools, relieve constipation and bloating and protect from colon damage. However, many patients don't get enough amounts of dietary fiber per day as many of them are high in potassium or phosphorus. Fortunately, there are some good dietary fiber sources for CKD patients that have lower amounts of these minerals compared to others.

Vitamins/Minerals

Our systems, according to medical research, need at least 13 vitamins and minerals to keep our cells fully active and healthy. Patients with renal disease though are more likely to be depleted by water-soluble vitamins like B-complex and Vitamin C, as a result, or limited fluid consumption. Therefore, supplementation with these vitamins along with a renal diet program should help cover any possible vitamin deficiencies. Supplementation of fat-soluble vitamins like vitamins A, K, and E may be avoided as they can quickly build up in the system and turn toxic.

Fluids

When you are in an advanced stage of renal disease, fluid can quickly build-up and lead to problems. While it is important to keep your system well hydrated, you should avoid minerals like potassium and sodium which can trigger further fluid build-up and cause a host of other symptoms.

Nutrients You Need To Avoid

Salt or sodium is known for being one of the most important ingredients that the renal diet prohibits its use. This ingredient, although simple, can badly and strongly affect your body and especially the kidneys. Any excess of sodium can't be easily filtered because of the failing condition of the kidneys. A large build-up of sodium can cause catastrophic results on your body. Potassium and Phosphorus are also prohibited for kidney patients depending on the stage of kidney disease.

Adopting a New Lifestyle to Minimize Your Kidney Problems

When you are recovering from acute renal failure or when you are on a renal failure diet, then your doctor or dietician would recommend a particular diet that would help you in limiting the stress on your kidneys. Your dietician would analyze and depending upon your current situation would suggest a diet that would reduce the pressure on your kidneys. Here are certain lifestyle changes that would help you in the recovery process and also help you to have healthy kidneys.

You should opt for foods that have a low level of potassium or no potassium at all. Foods rich in potassium include bananas, spinach, tomatoes, oranges and even potatoes. You can instead consume foods that have a low level of potassium in them like apples, cabbage, grapes, strawberries and green beans as well. You should avoid products that have added salt in them. You should cut down on the amount of sodium that you consume on a daily basis and this can be done by simply avoiding packed and canned foods, even frozen foods, you should also avoid processed meats as well as cheeses. Phosphorus is generally found in dairy products like milk, cheese and butter. It is also present in beans and nuts. You will need to reduce the amount of phosphorus that you consume because this weakens your bones and also cause skin irritation. Once your kidneys start recovering, your diet would change but that doesn't mean that you should stop eating healthy foods.

You should reduce or eliminate emotional stress. Quit smoking, alcohol consumption or any drugs not prescribed by a doctor.

Chapter 3: Shake and Drinks Recipes

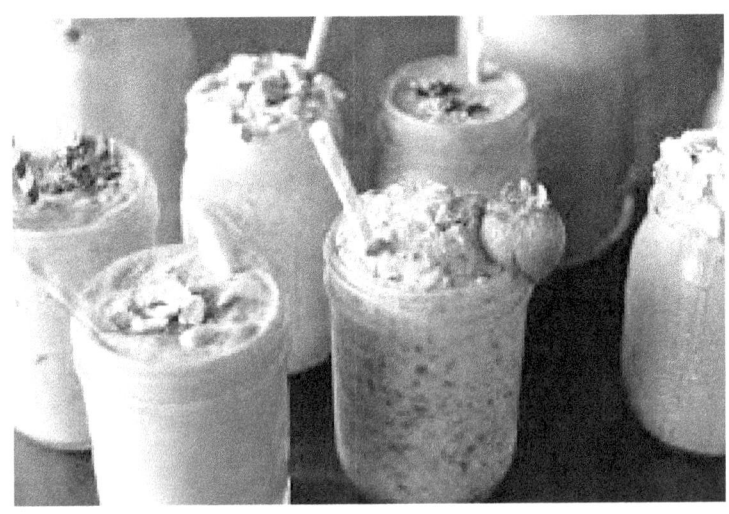

Blackberry Sage Water

Preparation Time: 15 minutes
Cooking Time: 0 minutes
Servings: 8
Ingredients:
15 medium fresh sage leaves
2 teaspoons stevia
1 cup boiling water
6 oz. fresh blackberries
Directions:
Add the sage leaves, stevia, blackberries, and water to a blender jug.
Blend well, then strain and refrigerate to chill.
Serve.
Nutrition:
Calories 24
Total Fat 0.3g

Saturated Fat 0.1g
Cholesterol 0mg
Sodium 1mg
Carbohydrate 2.9g
Dietary Fiber 1.6g
Sugars 1.9g
Protein 0.4g
Calcium 28mg
Phosphorous 13mg
Potassium 48mg

Berry Milk Smoothie

Preparation Time: 10 minutes
Cooking Time: 0 minutes
Servings: 1
Ingredients:
½ cup fresh blueberries
1 medium cucumber, peeled and sliced
½ cup fresh strawberries
½ cup almond milk
Directions:
First, begin by mixing all the ingredients into a blender jug.
Pulse it for 30 seconds until well blended.
Serve chilled.
Nutrition:
Calories 170
Total Fat 1.8g
Saturated Fat 0.2g
Cholesterol 0mg
Sodium 50mg
Carbohydrate 24.7g
Dietary Fiber 4.7g
Sugars 12.7g
Protein 3.2g
Calcium 70mg
Phosphorous 19mg
Potassium 243mg

Apple-Cinnamon Water

Preparation Time: 10 minutes
Cooking Time: 5 minutes
Servings: 8
Ingredients:
½ gallon water, filtered
3 apples, sliced
3 cinnamon sticks
Directions:
Add the water, apple slices, and cinnamon into a blender.

Pour this apple mixture into a suitable pot and cook for about 5 minutes.

Strain the apple-water and allow it to cool.

Serve.

Nutrition:
Calories 46
Total Fat 0.2g
Saturated Fat 0g
Cholesterol 0mg
Sodium 8mg
Total Carbohydrate 12.2g
Dietary Fiber 2.5g
Sugars 8.7g
Protein 0.3g
Calcium 16mg
Phosphorous 36 mg
Potassium 96mg

Caramel Latte

Preparation Time: 10 minutes
Cooking Time: 0 minutes
Servings: 1
Ingredients:

1/2 cup milk

1 tablespoon brown Swerve

1 tablespoon caramel topping

1 tablespoon caramel sauce

1/4 teaspoon vanilla extract

1 cup coffee

Directions:

Heat the milk in a 1-quart saucepan over moderate heat and add the Swerve, vanilla extract, and coffee.

Cook this latte up to a boil then pour into the serving mug.

Top it with caramel and sauce.

Enjoy.

Nutrition:

Calories 217

Total Fat 4.3g

Saturated Fat 2.8g

Cholesterol 15mg

Sodium 166mg

Carbohydrate 32.8g

Dietary Fiber 0.2g

Sugars 16.4g

Protein 4.6g

Calcium 168mg

Phosphorous 41mg

Potassium 217mg

Strawberry Smoothie

Preparation Time: 10 minutes
Cooking Time: 0 minutes
Servings: 1
Ingredients:
3/4 cup fresh strawberries
1/2 cup liquid egg whites, pasteurized
1/2 cup ice
Directions:
First, begin by putting everything into a blender jug.
Pulse it for 30 seconds until well blended.
Serve chilled.
Nutrition:
Calories 146
Total Fat 0.3g
Saturated Fat 0g
Cholesterol 0mg
Sodium 205mg
Carbohydrate 11.6g
Dietary Fiber 2.2g
Sugars 6.2g
Protein 14.1g
Calcium 21mg
Phosphorous 121mg
Potassium 166mg

Watermelon Mint Drink

Preparation Time: 10 minutes
Cooking Time: 0 minutes
Servings: 2
Ingredients:
6 cups seedless watermelon, cubed
The juice of 2 limes
1 cup of water
Directions:
First, begin by putting everything into a blender jug.
Pulse it for 30 seconds until well blended.
Serve chilled.
Nutrition:
Calories 148
Total Fat 0.6g
Saturated Fat 0.3g
Cholesterol 0mg
Sodium 11mg
Carbohydrate 38g
Dietary Fiber 2g
Sugars 28.7g
Protein 2.9g
Calcium 41mg
Phosphorous 24mg
Potassium 559mg

Beet Carrot Juice

Preparation Time: 10 minutes
Cooking Time: 0 minutes
Servings: 2
Ingredients:
1 medium beet, peeled and quartered

1 medium apple, peeled, cored and quartered

1 tablespoon fresh ginger

3 whole carrots, rinsed and peeled

½ cup apple juice

Directions:
Pass the beet, apple, ginger, and carrot through a juicer, one after another.

Pour the mix of the juices with the apple juice into two serving glasses and refrigerate to chill.

Serve.

Nutrition:
Calories 155

Total Fat 0.5g

Saturated Fat 0.1g

Cholesterol 0mg

Sodium 106mg

Carbohydrate 38.3g

Dietary Fiber 6.4g

Sugars 26.2g

Protein 2.2g

Calcium 47mg

Phosphorous 56mg

Potassium 663mg

Cinnamon Egg Smoothie

Preparation Time: 12 minutes
Cooking Time: 0 minutes
Servings: 2
Ingredients:
1/2 teaspoon ground cinnamon
1 teaspoon stevia
1/8 teaspoon vanilla extract
8 oz. egg white, pasteurized
3 tablespoons whipped topping
Directions:
Mix the stevia, egg whites, cinnamon, and vanilla in a mixer. Serve with whipped topping.
Enjoy.
Nutrition:
Calories 95
Total Fat 1.2g
Saturated Fat 0.6g
Cholesterol 3mg
Sodium 120mg
Carbohydrate 3.1g
Dietary Fiber 0.3g
Sugars 0.8g
Protein 12.5g
Calcium 18mg
Phosphorous 185mg
Potassium 194mg

Pineapple Sorbet Smoothie

Preparation Time: 15 minutes
Cooking Time: 0 minutes
Servings: 1
Ingredients:
3/4 cup pineapple sorbet
1 scoop protein powder
1/2 cup water
2 ice cubes, optional
Directions:
First, begin by putting everything into a blender jug.
Pulse it for 30 seconds until well blended.
Serve chilled.
Nutrition:
Calories 180
Total Fat 1g
Saturated Fat 0.5g
Cholesterol 40mg
Sodium 86mg
Carbohydrate 30.5g
Dietary Fiber 0g
Sugars 28g
Protein 13g
Calcium 9mg
Phosphorous 164mg
Potassium 111mg

Vanilla Fruit Smoothie

Preparation Time: 15 minutes
Cooking Time: 0 minutes
Servings: 2
Ingredients:
2 oz. mango, peeled and cubed
2 oz. strawberries
2 oz. avocado flesh, cubed
2 oz. banana, peeled
2 scoops of protein powder
1 cup cold water
1 cup crushed ice

Directions:
First, begin by putting everything into a blender jug.
Pulse it for 30 seconds until well blended.
Serve chilled.

Nutrition:
Calories 228
Total Fat 7.6g
Saturated Fat 2.1g
Cholesterol 65mg
Sodium 58mg
Total Carbohydrate 19g
Dietary Fiber 3.6g
Sugars 9.8g
Protein 23.4g
Calcium 112mg
Phosphorous 216 mg
Potassium 504mg

Protein Berry Smoothie

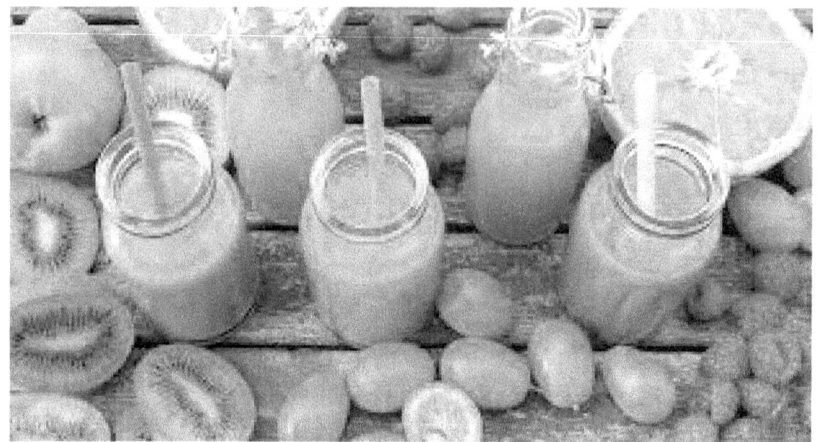

Preparation Time: 12 minutes
Cooking Time: 0 minutes
Servings: 2
Ingredients:
4 oz. water
1 cup frozen mixed berries
2 ice cubes
1 teaspoon blueberry essence
2 scoops whey protein powder
Directions:
First, begin by putting everything into a blender jug.
Pulse it for 30 seconds until well blended.
Serve chilled.
Nutrition:
Calories 248
Total Fat 11.4g
Saturated Fat 6.7g
Cholesterol 98mg
Sodium 67mg

Carbohydrate 13.3g
Dietary Fiber 2.5g
Sugars 6.1g
Protein 23.3g
Calcium 132mg
Phosphorous 152mg
Potassium 296mg

Protein Peach Smoothie

Preparation Time: 12 minutes
Cooking Time: 0 minutes
Servings: 1
Ingredients:

1/2 cup ice

2 tablespoons egg whites, pasteurized

3/4 cup fresh peaches

1 teaspoon stevia

Directions:

First, begin by putting everything into a blender jug.

Pulse it for 30 seconds until well blended.

Serve chilled.

Nutrition:

Calories 195

Total Fat 0.3g

Saturated Fat 0g

Cholesterol 0mg

Sodium 347mg

Carbohydrate 17g

Dietary Fiber 1.7g

Sugars 14.2g

Protein 24.1g

Calcium 25mg

Phosphorous 233mg

Potassium 526mg

Cranberry Cucumber Smoothie

Preparation Time: 10 minutes
Cooking Time: 0 minutes
Servings: 1
Ingredients:

1 cup frozen cranberries

1 medium cucumber, peeled and sliced

1 stalk of celery

1 teaspoon lime juice

Directions:

First, begin by putting everything into a blender jug. Pulse it for 30 seconds until well blended. Serve chilled.

Nutrition:

Calories 119

Total Fat 0.4g

Saturated Fat 0.1g

Cholesterol 0mg

Sodium 21mg

Carbohydrate 25.1g

Dietary Fiber 6g

Sugars 10g

Protein 2.3g

Calcium 79mg

Phosphorous 184mg

Potassium 325mg

Raspberry Smoothie

Preparation Time: 12 minutes
Cooking Time: 0 minutes
Servings: 2
Ingredients:
1 cup frozen raspberries
1 medium peach, pitted, sliced
½ cup tofu
1 tablespoon honey
1 cup milk
Directions:
First, begin by putting everything into a blender jug.
Pulse it for 30 seconds until well blended.
Serve chilled.
Nutrition:
Calories 223
Total Fat 2.7g
Saturated Fat 0.3g
Cholesterol 0mg
Sodium 99mg
Carbohydrate 49.9g
Dietary Fiber 7.2g
Sugars 43.1g
Protein 3.6g
Calcium 176mg
Phosphorous 95mg
Potassium 426mg

Citrus Pineapple Shake

Preparation Time: 15 minutes
Cooking Time: 0 minutes
Servings: 2
Ingredients:
1/2 cup pineapple juice
1/2 cup almond milk
1 cup orange sherbet
1/2 cup egg, pasteurized
Directions:
Pour the almond milk, pineapple juice, sherbet, and egg into the blender.

Blend well for 1 minute then refrigerate to chill.

Serve.
Nutrition:
Calories 242
Total Fat 8.2g
Saturated Fat 2.8g
Cholesterol 227mg
Sodium 155mg
Carbohydrate 33g
Dietary Fiber 1.1g
Sugars 26.2g
Protein 8.9g
Calcium 80mg
Phosphorous 121mg
Potassium 234mg

Pineapple Smoothie

Preparation Time: 15 minutes
Cooking Time: 0 minutes
Servings: 2
Ingredients:
3/4 cup pineapple sherbet
1 scoop protein powder
1/2 cup water
2 ice cubes
Directions:
Add the water, pineapple sherbet, protein powder, and ice to a blender.

Blend the pineapple smoothie for 1 minute.

Serve.
Nutrition:
Calories 91
Total Fat 0.6g
Saturated Fat 0.2g
Cholesterol 7mg
Sodium 36mg
Carbohydrate 10.4g
Dietary Fiber 0g
Sugars 8g
Protein 11.9g
Calcium 208mg
Phosphorous 49mg
Potassium 25mg

Hazelnut Coffee

Preparation Time: 15 minutes
Cooking Time: 0 minutes
Servings: 2
Ingredients:
4 cups brewed coffee
8 teaspoons hazelnut syrup
4 tablespoons almond milk
8 cinnamon sticks

Directions:
Begin by brewing the coffee in a coffee maker, then pour it into the 4 small serving cups.

Add 1 tablespoon almond milk, 2 teaspoons hazelnut syrup, and 2 cinnamon sticks to each mug.

Serve.

Nutrition:
Calories 65
Total Fat 4.5g
Saturated Fat 0.7g
Cholesterol 3mg
Sodium 24mg
Carbohydrate 4.4g
Dietary Fiber 1.8g
Sugars 1.7g
Protein 2.6g
Calcium 76mg
Phosphorous 73mg
Potassium 302mg

Lemon Piña Colada

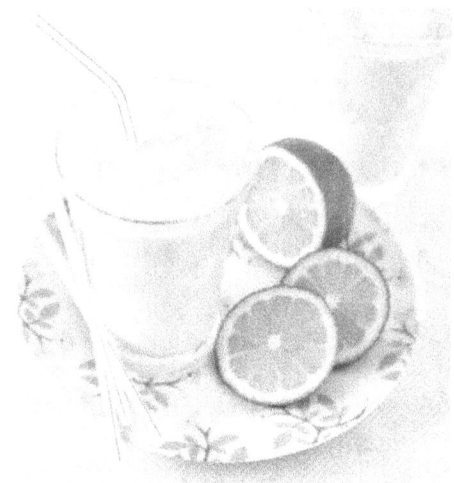

Preparation Time: 15 minutes
Cooking Time: 0 minutes
Servings: 1
Ingredients:
6 oz. pineapple juice

1 oz. lemon-lime juice

1 oz. protein powder

1/2 cup crushed ice

2 slices fresh pineapple

Directions:
Put the protein powder, pineapple juice, and ice into a blender jug.

Pour the piña colada mixture into the serving glasses.

Top the Piña Coladas with lemon-lime juice.

Garnish with pineapple slices.

Serve.

Nutrition:
Calories 227
Total Fat 2.2g
Saturated Fat 1.1g
Cholesterol 59mg
Sodium 60mg
Carbohydrate 31.3g
Dietary Fiber 1g
Sugars 22.5g
Protein 21.3g
Calcium 121mg
Phosphorous 94mg
Potassium 462mg

Blueberry Apple Blast

Preparation Time: 10 minutes
Cooking Time: 0 minutes
Servings: 2
Ingredients:
1 cup frozen blueberries
6 tablespoons vanilla protein powder
8 ice cubes
14 oz. apple juice
Directions:
First, begin by putting everything into a blender jug.
Pulse it for 30 seconds until well blended.
Serve chilled.
Nutrition:
Calories 260
Total Fat 2.3g
Saturated Fat 1g
Cholesterol 65mg
Sodium 71mg
Carbohydrate 38.3g
Dietary Fiber 2g
Sugars 8.1g
Protein 23g
Calcium 113mg
Phosphorous 105mg
Potassium 495mg

Allspice Cider

Preparation Time: 12 minutes
Cooking Time: 0 minutes
Servings: 8
Ingredients:

8 cups apple cider

3 cinnamon sticks

1/4 teaspoon whole cloves

1/4 teaspoon ground allspice

Directions:

Add the cider, cinnamon sticks, allspice, and cloves to a slow cooker.

Cook this apple cider mixture for 1 hour on low heat.

Strain and serve.

Nutrition:

Calories 118

Total Fat 0.3g

Saturated Fat 0.1g

Cholesterol 0mg

Sodium 8mg

Carbohydrate 29.3g

Dietary Fiber 0.4g

Sugars 27g

Protein 0.2g

Calcium 21mg

Phosphorous 124mg

Potassium 298mg

Chapter 4: Seafood Recipes

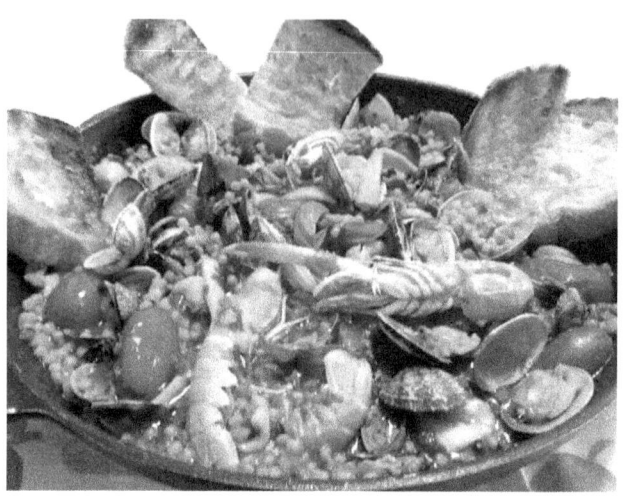

Shrimp Paella

Preparation Time: 5 minutes
Cooking Time: 10 minutes
Servings: 2

Ingredients:
1 cup cooked brown rice
1 chopped red onion
1 tsp. paprika
1 chopped garlic clove
1 tbsp. olive oil
6 oz. frozen cooked shrimp
1 deseeded and sliced chili pepper
1 tbsp. oregano

Directions:
Heat the olive oil in a large pan on medium-high heat.
Add the onion and garlic and sauté for 2-3 minutes until soft.

Now add the shrimp and sauté for a further 5 minutes or until hot through.

Now add the herbs, spices, chili and rice with 1/2 cup boiling water.

Stir until everything is warm and the water has been absorbed.

Plate up and serve.

Nutrition:

Calories 221

Protein 17 g

Carbs 31 g

Fat 8 g

Sodium (Na) 235 mg

Potassium (K) 176 mg

Phosphorus 189 mg

Salmon & Pesto Salad

Preparation Time: 5 minutes
Cooking Time: 15 minutes
Servings: 2
Ingredients:

1 minced garlic clove

½ cup fresh arugula

¼ cup extra virgin olive oil

½ cup fresh basil

1 tsp. black pepper

4 oz. skinless salmon fillet

1 tbsp. coconut oil

½ juiced lemon

2 sliced radishes

½ cup iceberg lettuce

1 tsp. black pepper

Directions:

Prepare the pesto by blending all the ingredients for the pesto in a food processor or by grinding with a pestle and mortar. Set aside.

Add a skillet to the stove on medium-high heat and melt the coconut oil.

Add the salmon to the pan.

Cook for 7-8 minutes and turn over.

Cook for a further 3-4 minutes or until cooked through.

Remove fillets from the skillet and allow to rest.

Mix the lettuce and the radishes and squeeze over the juice of ½ lemon.

Flake the salmon with a fork and mix through the salad.

Toss to coat and sprinkle with a little black pepper to serve.

Nutrition:
Calories 221
Protein 13 g
Carbs 1 g
Fat 34 g
Sodium (Na) 80 mg
Potassium (K) 119 mg
Phosphorus 158 mg

Baked Fennel & Garlic Sea Bass

Preparation Time: 5 minutes
Cooking Time: 15 minutes
Servings: 2
Ingredients:

1 lemon

½ sliced fennel bulb

6 oz. sea bass fillets

1 tsp. black pepper

2 garlic cloves

Directions:

Preheat the oven to 375°F/Gas Mark 5.

Sprinkle black pepper over the Sea Bass.

Slice the fennel bulb and garlic cloves.

Add 1 salmon fillet and half the fennel and garlic to one sheet of baking paper or tin foil.

Squeeze in 1/2 lemon juices.

Repeat for the other fillet.

Fold and add to the oven for 12-15 minutes or until fish is thoroughly cooked through.

Meanwhile, add boiling water to your couscous, cover and allow to steam.

Serve with your choice of rice or salad.

Nutrition:

Calories 221

Protein 14 g

Carbs 3 g

Fat 2 g

Sodium (Na) 119 mg

Potassium (K) 398 mg

Phosphorus 149 mg

Lemon, Garlic & Cilantro Tuna and Rice

Preparation Time: 5 minutes
Cooking Time: 0 minutes
Servings: 2
Ingredients:

½ cup arugula

1 tbsp. extra virgin olive oil

1 cup cooked rice

1 tsp. black pepper

¼ finely diced red onion

1 juiced lemon

3 oz. canned tuna

2 tbsps. Chopped fresh cilantro

Directions:

Mix the olive oil, pepper, cilantro and red onion in a bowl.

Stir in the tuna, cover and leave in the fridge for as long as possible (if you can) or serve immediately.

When ready to eat, serve up with the cooked rice and arugula!

Nutrition:

Calories 221

Protein 11 g

Carbs 26 g

Fat 7 g

Sodium (Na) 143 mg

Potassium (K) 197 mg

Phosphorus 182 mg

Salmon and Sweet Potato Chowder

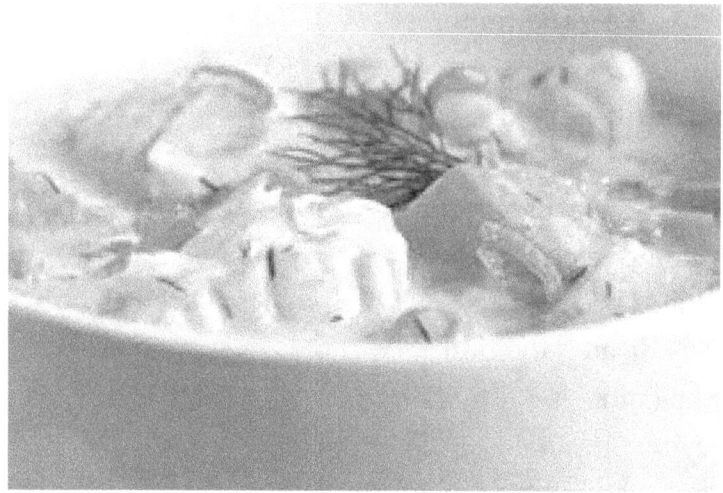

Preparation Time: 15 minutes
Cooking Time: 4 hours
Servings: 4
Ingredients:
1 tbsp. Butter
1 minced clove of Garlic
1 chopped Onion
2 tsp. Dill Weed
3 tbsp. o all-purpose Flour
Ground Black Pepper
2 cups Milk
2 cups Sweet Potatoes (diced)
2 cups Chicken Broth
1 ½ cups Corn Kernels
1 tsp. Lemon Zest
12 ounces sliced Salmon Fillets
3 tbsp. Lemon Juice

Directions:

Sauté pepper, dill, garlic and onion in butter in a pan.

Add in the flour and cook for 2 minutes.

Pour broth and then milk to the pan. Simmer.

Pour the mixture to the slow cooker and add the sweet potatoes.

Cook on "low" for 4 hrs.

Add in the salmon and cook again on "low" for 20 more minutes.

Now, stir in the lemon zest, lemon juice along with the pepper.

Serve hot in heated bowls.

Nutrition:

391 Calories

27 g Total Fat

94 mg Cholesterol

320 mg Sodium

39 mg Carbohydrates

7 g Dietary Fiber

37 g Protein

Sesame Salmon Fillets

Preparation Time: 15 minutes
Cooking Time: 30 minutes
Servings: 2
Ingredients:
2 tbsp. Sesame Oil

¼ tsp. Sea Salt

¼ tsp. Black Pepper (cracked)

1 tbsp. Vinegar

4 tsp. Sesame Seeds (black)

¼ tsp. Ginger (ground)

4 skinless Salmon fillets

Directions:
Coat the slow cooker with oil. Set the cooker on "high".

Place the salmon in the cooker. Drizzle the sesame seeds, pepper, salt and ginger on the salmon.

Turn after 3 minutes and repeat the procedure.

Add vinegar and cook on "high" for 20 minutes.

Transfer the salmon to a plate. Serve immediately

Nutrition:
319 Calories

21 g Total Fats

81 mg Cholesterol

204 mg Sodium

31 g Carbohydrates

1 g Dietary Fiber

31 g Protein

Peppered Balsamic Cod

Preparation Time: 10 minutes
Cooking Time: 2 hours
Servings: 4
Ingredients:

1 1/2 pounds cod filets

2 teaspoons olive oil

1 teaspoon lemon zest

1/2 teaspoon cracked black peppercorns

2 tablespoons balsamic vinegar, reduced to a syrup

Directions:

Cut a piece of foil large enough to wrap completely around the fish, or cut 4 smaller pieces to wrap the fish into individual packets. Brush the foil with 1 teaspoon of the oil. Arrange the fish in the center of the foil and brush with the remaining oil. Season evenly with the lemon zest and pepper. Drizzle with the balsamic vinegar. Fold the foil completely around the fish and crimp the edges to seal the package(s) completely.

Set the package in the slow cooker, cover with a lid, and cook on HIGH for 2 hours, or until the fish is completely cooked.

Serve at once.

Nutrition:

Calories 201

Total Fat 5g

Saturated Fat 1g

Cholesterol 101mg

Sodium 121mg

Total Carbohydrates 1g

Dietary Fiber 1g

Protein 39g

Sugars 1g

Seafood Gumbo

Preparation Time: 25 minutes
Cooking Time: 5 hours
Servings: 6
Ingredients:
2 teaspoons olive oil
1/4 cup minced turkey ham (low sodium)
2 stalks celery, sliced
1 medium onion, sliced
1 green bell pepper, chopped
2 cloves garlic, minced
2 cups chicken broth (low sodium)
1 (14-ounce) can diced tomatoes, including juices
1 teaspoon Worcestershire sauce
1/4 teaspoon kosher salt
1 teaspoon dried thyme
1-pound shrimp (16/20), cleaned
1 pound fresh or frozen crabmeat, picked to remove cartilage
1 (10-ounce) package frozen okra, thawed

Directions:

Heat the oil in a sauté pan over medium-high heat. Add the ham and cook until crisp. With a slotted spoon, transfer the ham to a slow cooker.

Add the celery, onion, green pepper, and garlic to the sauté pan and cook over medium heat, stirring frequently, until the vegetables are tender, about 10 minutes. Transfer to the cooker and add the broth, tomatoes and their juices, Worcestershire, salt, and thyme.

Cover and cook on LOW for 4 hours. Add the shrimp, crabmeat, and okra, and cook on HIGH for 20 minutes or until the shrimp is bright pink and firm.

Serve at once in heated soup bowls.

Nutrition:
Calories 155
Total Fat 5g
Saturated Fat 3g
Cholesterol 207mg
Sodium 313mg
Total Carbohydrates 16g
Dietary Fiber 5g
Protein 22g
Sugars 2g

Salmon Chowder with Sweet Potatoes and Corn

Preparation Time: 10 minutes
Cooking Time: 4 hours
Servings: 4
Ingredients:

1 tablespoon butter

1 onion, finely chopped

1 clove garlic, minced

2 teaspoons dill weed

Freshly ground black pepper

3 tablespoons all-purpose flour

2 cups chicken broth (low sodium)

2 cups milk ()

2 cups diced sweet potatoes

1 1/2 cups fresh or thawed frozen corn kernels

12 ounces salmon fillet, cut into chunks

1 teaspoon grated lemon zest

3 tablespoons lemon juice

Directions:

Melt the butter in a saucepan over medium heat. Add the onion, garlic, dill, and a pinch of pepper; sauté, stirring frequently, until the onion is tender. Add the flour and stir until thick and pasty, about 2 minutes. Whisk in the broth until there are no lumps, then stir in the milk, and bring to a simmer. Pour into the slow cooker and add the sweet potatoes and corn. Cover with a lid and cook on LOW for 4 hours, until the potatoes are very tender.

Stir in the salmon, replace the lid, and cook on LOW for 20 minutes, or until the salmon is cooked (145°F) and very hot. Stir in the lemon zest and season to taste with lemon juice and additional pepper.

Serve in heated soup bowls.

Nutrition:
Calories 391
Total Fat: 18g
Saturated Fat: 9g
Cholesterol: 94mg
Sodium 320mg
Total Carbohydrates: 39g
Dietary Fiber: 7g
Protein 37g
Sugars 17g

Mediterranean Fish Stew

Preparation Time: 15 minutes
Cooking Time: 4 hours
Servings: 6
Ingredients:
1 onion, sliced
1 leek, white and light green portion, sliced thin
4 cloves garlic, minced
1/2 cup dry white wine
1/4 cup water
4 bay leaves
1-piece orange peel, 2 inches, pith removed
1/2 teaspoon cracked black peppercorns
1 1/2 pounds haddock fillets
12 ounces shrimp (16/20), peeled and deveined
2 teaspoons extra-virgin olive oil for serving
2 tablespoons chopped parsley, flat leaf
Directions:
Make a bed of the onion, leek, and garlic in the slow cooker. Add the wine and water to the cooker. Scatter the bay leaves, orange peel, and peppercorns on top. Cover the cooker and cook on HIGH for 2 hours. Add the fish and the shrimp, replace the cover, and cook on HIGH for an additional 2 hours or until the fish is cooked through and the shrimps are bright pink and opaque. Remove and discard the bay leaves and orange peel.
Serve the fish and shrimp in heated soup bowls topped with the cooking liquid and vegetables. Drizzle with olive oil and garnish with parsley.
Nutrition:
Calories 207
Total Fat: 4g
Saturated Fat: 0g
Cholesterol: 168mg
Sodium 536mg
Total Carbohydrates: 5g
Dietary Fiber: 1g
Protein 32g
Sugars 0g

Tuna and Red Pepper Stew

Preparation Time: 15 minutes
Cooking Time: 4 hours
Servings: 6
Ingredients:
1 tablespoon olive oil
1 onion, chopped
1 garlic clove, minced
1/4 teaspoon red pepper flakes, or more to taste
1/2 cup dry white wine
1 (14-ounce) can diced tomatoes
1-pound baby red potatoes, scrubbed
1 teaspoon paprika
2 pounds tuna fillet
2 roasted red bell peppers, seeded and cut into strips
3 tablespoons chopped cilantro for garnish

Directions:
Combine the oil, onions, garlic, red pepper flakes, wine, tomatoes, and potatoes, in a slow cooker. Cover and cook on HIGH for 2 hours. Add the tuna and the roasted peppers, season with the paprika, and replace the cover. Continue to cook on HIGH for another 2 hours or until the tuna is fully cooked.

Serve at once, topped with the cilantro.

Nutrition:
Calories 107
Total Fat: 3g
Saturated Fat: 0g
Cholesterol: 8mg
Sodium 200mg
Total Carbohydrates: 15g
Dietary Fiber: 2g
Protein 5g
Sugars 0g

Sweet and Sour Shrimp

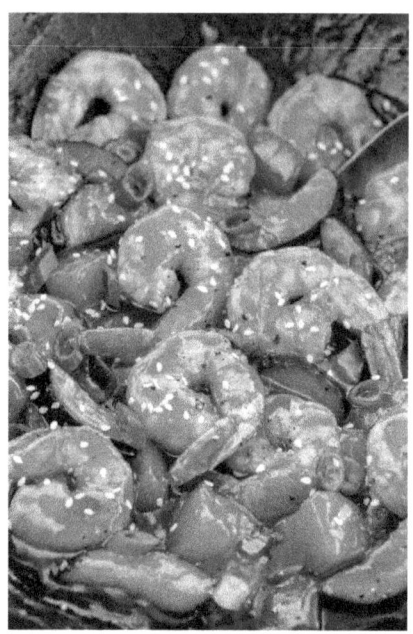

Preparation Time: 10 minutes
Cooking Time: 5 hours and 30 minutes
Servings: 3-4
Ingredients:
1 cup Chinese pea pods, thawed
1 14oz can pineapple chunks
2 tablespoons cornstarch
3 tbsp. sugar
1 cup chicken stock (see recipe)
½ cup reserved pineapple juice
1 tbsp. low-sodium soy sauce
½ tsp. ground ginger
1lb large cooked shrimp
2 tbsp. cider vinegar
1 cup of rice, cooked

Directions:

Place the pea pods and pineapple in a 4 to 6-quart slow cooker.

Blend the cornstarch and sugar with the chicken stock and pineapple juice and heat in a small saucepan until thickened.

Pour the sauce into the slow cooker and add the ginger and soy sauce.

Cover and cook on LOW for 3 to 4 hours.

Add the shrimp and vinegar and cook for a further 15 minutes.

Serve with the hot cooked rice.

Nutrition:

Calories 395

Fat 2g

Carbs 61g

Protein 33g

Fiber 5g

Potassium 796mg

Sodium 215 mg

Salmon with Caramelized Onions

Preparation Time: 20 minutes
Cooking Time: 6 hours
Servings: 6
Ingredients:
1lb salmon fillet, cut into small fillets
1 tbsp. extra-virgin olive oil
½ large onion, thinly sliced
¼ tsp. ground ginger
¼ tsp. dried dill
¼ tsp. low-sodium salt
¼ tsp. black pepper
½ lemon, thinly sliced

Directions:
Arrange the onions in the base of a 4 to 6-quart slow cooker.

Place each piece of salmon in an aluminum foil packet and sprinkle with spices and top with lemon slices.

Place the salmon packets on top of the onions in the slow cooker and cover.

Cook on LOW for 6 to 8 hours.

Serve the salmon on top of the onions.

Nutrition:
Calories 215

Fat 11g

Carbs 7g

Protein 24g

Fiber 2g

Potassium 520mg

Sodium 200mg

Slow Cooker Shrimp in Tomato Sauce

Preparation Time: 15 minutes
Cooking Time: 4 hours
Servings: 4
Ingredients:
1 14oz can of no-added sodium crushed tomatoes
1 6oz can of no-added salt tomato paste
1 garlic clove, minced
1 tsp. low-sodium salt
2 tsp. fresh basil, chopped
½ tsp. dried oregano
¼ tsp. freshly ground black pepper
½ tsp. crushed red pepper flakes
2 tbsp. fresh parsley, minced
1lb cooked shrimp, peeled and deveined
½ cup low-sodium Parmesan cheese, grated
4 cup cooked spaghetti

Directions:
Place the tomatoes, tomato paste, garlic, salt, basil, oregano, salt, black pepper, and crushed red pepper, into a 4 to 6-quart slow cooker. If using.

Cover and cook on LOW for 4 to 5 hours.

Add the shrimp and parsley and cook on HIGH for 10 minutes.

Serve the shrimp on top of the hot cooked pasta with low-sodium Parmesan cheese.

Nutrition:
Calories 509
Fat 5g
Carbs 69g
Protein 48g
Fiber 7g
Potassium 629mg
Sodium 400mg

Fisherman's Stew

Preparation Time: 20 minutes
Cooking Time: 6-8 hours
Servings: 8
Ingredients:
1 fillet of sea bass, cod or other white fish, cubed
1 dozen each large shrimp, scallops, mussels & clams
1 28 ounces no-added salt crushed tomatoes with juice
1 8oz no-added salt tomato sauce
½ cup onion, chopped
1 cup dry white wine
1/3 cup olive oil
3 garlic cloves, minced
½ cup parsley, chopped
1 green pepper, chopped
1 hot pepper, chopped
½ tsp. low sodium salt
1 tsp. thyme
2 tsp. basil
1 tsp. oregano
½ tsp. paprika
½ tsp. cayenne pepper

Directions:
Place all ingredients except seafood in a 4 to 6-quart slow cooker and cover.
Cook on LOW for 6 to 8 hours.
Add the fish about 30 minutes towards the end of the cooking time and turn up the heat to HIGH.

Nutrition:
Calories 434
Fat 16g
Carbs 27g
Protein 39g
Fiber 4g
Potassium 714mg
Sodium 378mg

Fish Chowder

Preparation Time: 15 minutes
Cooking Time: 6 hours
Servings: 6
Ingredients:
2lb white fish fillets, cut into 1-inch pieces
¼lb low-sodium bacon, diced
1 medium onion, chopped
4 medium red-skinned potatoes, peeled and cubed
2 cup water
1 low sodium salt
¼ tsp. black pepper
1 12oz can evaporated milk
Directions:
Fry the bacon in a skillet for a few minutes with the onion.
Add the bacon to the slow cooker with the remaining ingredients except for the evaporated milk.
Cover and cook on HIGH for 5 to 6 hours.
Add the milk during the last hour of cooking.
Nutrition:
Calories 311
Fat 13g
Carbs 27g
Protein 14g
Fiber 12g
Potassium 911mg
Sodium 600mg

Shrimp Creole

Preparation Time: 15 minutes
Cooking Time: 4 hours
Servings: 2-3
Ingredients:
1½ cup celery, diced
1¼ cup onion, chopped
1 cup bell pepper, chopped
1 8oz can no-added salt tomato sauce
1 28oz no-added salt can whole tomatoes
1 garlic clove, minced
½ tsp. low-sodium salt
½ tsp. salt-free Creole seasoning
¼ tsp. freshly ground black pepper
6 drops Tabasco sauce
1lb shrimp, deveined and shelled

Directions:
Place all the ingredients into a 3-quart slow cooker except the shrimp.
Cook 3 to 4 hours on high or 6 to 8 hours on low.
Add shrimp during last 30 minutes of cooking.
Serve over hot cooked rice

Nutrition:
Calories 388
Fat 3g
Carbs 42g
Protein 52g
Fiber 8g
Potassium 874mg
Sodium 600mg

Baked Fish

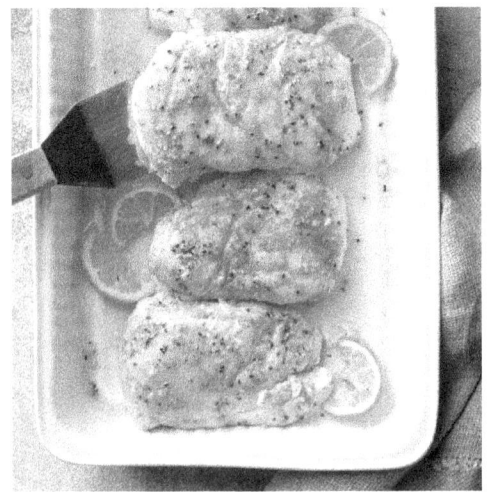

Preparation Time: 15 minutes
Cooking Time: 25 hours
Servings: 4
Ingredients:
Cod fillets – 1lb/0,45gr
Olive oil – 2tbsp.
Ground cumin – ½ tsp.
Ground rosemary – ½ tsp.
Black pepper – ½ tsp.
Directions:
Preheat the oven to 350°F (176°C) and in the meantime turn cod fillet several times in olive oil, then sprinkle with spices
Place fillets in a baking dish and bake for 20 to 25 minutes
Nutrition:
Calories – 171
Carbohydrate – 0g
Protein – 20g
Sodium – 69mg
Potassium – 338mg
Phosphorus – 204mg
Dietary fiber – 0.2g
Fat – 10g

Creamy Tuna

Preparation Time: 15 minutes
Cooking Time: 10-20 minutes
Servings: 4
Ingredients:

Mayonnaise – ¾ cup

Vinegar – 2tbsp.

Shell macaroni (cooked) – 1 ½ cups

Tuna (drained) – 1 can (water-packed or unsalted)

Peas (cooked) – ½ cup

Celery (chopped) – ½ cup

Dried dill – 1tbsp.

Directions:

Mix mayo, vinegar, and macaroni in a large bowl add other ingredients

Cover and chill

Nutrition:

Calories – 415

Carbohydrate – 15g

Protein – 12g

Sodium – 258mg

Potassium – 175mg

Phosphorus – 116mg

Dietary fiber – 2.2g

Fat – 15.5g

Savory Salmon Dip

Preparation Time: 20 minutes
Cooking Time: 1 hour and 10 minutes
Servings: 12
Ingredients:
Salmon (skinless, boneless) – 1lb/0.45kg
Smoked paprika – 2tsp.
Cream cheese – 1 cup
Capers – ¼ cup
Lemon juice – ¼ cup
Lemon zest – 1tsp.
Red onions (diced) – 2tbsp.
Ground black pepper – 1tsp.
Parsley (chopped) – 1tbsp.
Water – 2 cups

Directions:
Over medium-high heat poach salmon with 1tsp. of smoked paprika and 2 cups of water for 4 to 6 minutes

Remove from the heat and let sit for 30 minutes

Combine other ingredients

Add salmon to the bowl with other ingredients and chill for 20 to 30 minutes before serving

Nutrition:
Calories – 133
Carbohydrate – 2g
Protein – 10g
Sodium – 147mg
Potassium – 259mg
Phosphorus – 110mg
Dietary fiber – 0mg
Fat – 9g

Chapter 5: Poultry Recipes

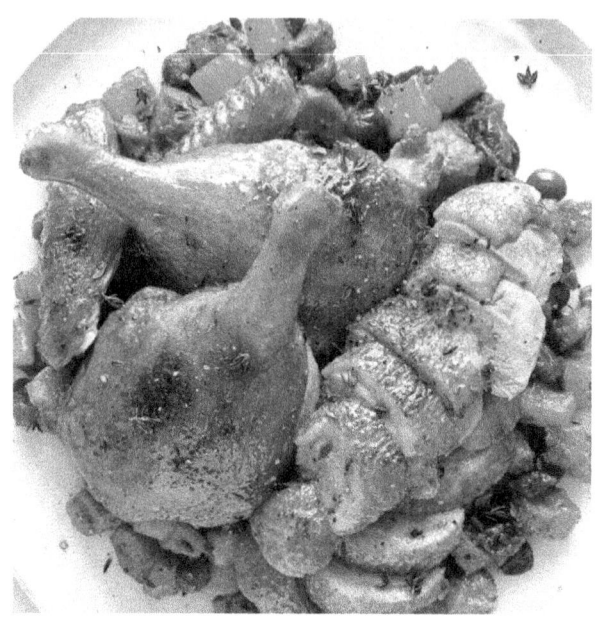

Lemon & Herb Chicken Wraps

Preparation Time: 5 minutes
Cooking Time: 30 minutes
Servings: 4
Ingredients:
4 oz. skinless and sliced chicken breasts
½ sliced red bell pepper
1 lemon
4 large iceberg lettuce leaves
1 tbsp. olive oil
2 tbsps. Finely chopped fresh cilantro
¼ tsp. black pepper
Directions:
Preheat the oven to 375°F/Gas Mark 5.
Mix the oil, juice of ½ lemon, cilantro and black pepper.

Marinate the chicken in the oil marinade, cover and leave in the fridge for as long as possible.

Wrap the chicken in parchment paper, drizzling over the remaining marinade.

Place in the oven in an oven dish for 25-30 minutes or until chicken is thoroughly cooked through and white inside.

Divide the sliced bell pepper and layer onto each lettuce leaf.

Divide the chicken onto each lettuce leaf and squeeze over the remaining lemon juice to taste.

Season with a little extra black pepper if desired.

Wrap and enjoy!

Nutrition:

Calories 200

Protein 9 g

Carbs 5 g

Fat 13 g

Sodium (Na) 25 mg

Potassium (K) 125 mg

Phosphorus 81 mg

Carrot & Ginger Chicken Noodles

Preparation Time: 5 minutes
Cooking Time: 10 minutes
Servings: 4
Ingredients:
1 sliced green onion
2 tsps. grated fresh ginger
4 oz. skinless sliced chicken breasts
1 lime
1 minced garlic clove
1 cup cooked rice noodles
1 tsp. coconut oil
1 peeled and grated carrot

Directions:
Heat a wok or large pan over medium-high heat.

Add the coconut oil to a pan and once melted, add the sliced chicken and brown for 4-5 minutes.

Now add the ginger and garlic and sauté for 4-5 minutes.

Add the green onion, carrot and lime juice to the wok.

Add the cooked noodles to the wok and toss until hot through.

Serve piping hot and enjoy.

Nutrition:
Calories 187
Protein 11 g
Carbs 25 g
Fat 5 g
Sodium (Na) 39 mg
Potassium (K) 91 mg
Phosphorus 178 mg

Rosemary and Lemon Chicken with Eggplant

Preparation Time: 10 minutes
Cooking Time: 40 minutes
Servings: 4
Ingredients:
6 oz skinless chicken breasts
1/2 white onion, roughly chopped
2 garlic cloves, chopped
1 cup cubed eggplant
2 tbsp. rosemary, fresh or dried
A pinch of black pepper
1/4 cup water
1 tbsp. extra virgin olive oil
1 tbsp. balsamic vinegar
1/2 lemon
1 tbsp. fresh basil

Directions:
Preheat the oven to 375°F/190°C/Gas Mark 5.
Add the chicken, onion, garlic and eggplant to a lined baking tray and sprinkle over the rosemary and black pepper.
Pour over the water, olive oil and balsamic vinegar, so that the chicken and vegetables are sitting in a shallow bath.
Add 1/2 lemon to the baking tray for flavor.
Bake in the oven for 35-40 minutes or until the chicken is completely cooked through.
Serve the chicken and eggplant with a sprinkle of freshly torn basil and a little extra black pepper to serve.

Nutrition:
Calories: 121
Fat: 5g;
Carbohydrates: 6g
Phosphorus: 108mg
Potassium: 231mg
Sodium: 210mg
Protein: 13g

Parsley and Turkey Cabbage Wraps

Preparation Time: 15 minutes
Cooking Time: 45 minutes
Servings: 4
Ingredients:
4 medium green cabbage leaves
7 oz. ground lean turkey
1/2 onion, finely diced
1 medium red bell pepper, finely diced
1 tbsp. parsley
1 tsp. cracked black pepper
Directions:
Preheat the oven to 375°F/190°C/Gas Mark 5.
Carefully pull off the cabbage leaves from the cabbage, wash and leave intact.
Mix the rest of the ingredients in a bowl and divide into quarters.
Take a cabbage leaf and add a quarter of the mixture to the end of the leaf.
Roll from the stuffing end until you've wrapped the leaf around the stuffing.
Pierce through the centre with a toothpick so that the wraps stay together.
Repeat for the rest of the mixture.
Add the cabbage rolls to an oven dish and pour 1/2 cup water into the bottom, cover with a lid and bake for 45 minutes or until turkey is completely cooked through.
Remove from the oven and serve.
Nutrition:
Calories: 106
Fat: 6g
Carbohydrates: 4g
Phosphorus: 105g
Potassium: 206mg
Sodium: 32mg
Protein: 9g

Turkey and Couscous Stuffed Bell Peppers

Preparation Time: 15 minutes
Cooking Time: 40 minutes
Servings: 4
Ingredients:
1/2 cup dried couscous
2 small red bell peppers
4 oz. lean ground turkey
1/2 red onion, finely diced
1 clove garlic, minced
1/2 tsp. cayenne pepper
1 tbsp. parsley
1 tsp. black pepper
1/2 lime

Directions:
Preheat the oven to 350°f/170°c/Gas Mark 4.
In a heatproof bowl or dish, pour 1/2 cup boiling water over the couscous, cover and allow to steam for 3 minutes or according to package directions
Meanwhile, slice each pepper in half lengthways.
Remove the seeds from the middle of the bell peppers and layer onto a baking tray.
Combine the turkey mince with the onion, garlic, herbs and spices.
Stuff the peppers with the mixture.
Add to the oven for 30-40 minutes or until turkey is cooked through.
Serve with a side of couscous and a squeeze of fresh lime.

Nutrition:
Calories: 143
Fat: 8g
Carbohydrates: 20g
Phosphorus: 79mg
Potassium: 190mg
Sodium: 22mg
Protein: 8g

Zesty Caribbean Chicken

Preparation Time: 5 minutes
Cooking Time: 40 minutes
Servings: 4
Ingredients:
1 tbsp. coconut oil
1 tbsp. honey
1 tbsp. mustard
2 tsp. curry powder
1 garlic clove, minced
1 tbsp. jamaican spice blend/allspice
4x small skinless chicken thighs
3/4 cup white rice
1/2 cup fresh or frozen green peas
1 lime

Directions:
Preheat the oven to 350°f/170°c/Gas Mark 4.

Allow coconut oil to melt by warming in your hands or for a few seconds in a pan over the stove.

In a separate bowl, prepare marinade by mixing melted coconut oil, honey, mustard, garlic, and spices.

Pour over the chicken into a baking dish.

Place in the oven for 35-40 minutes.

Meanwhile, prepare your rice: bring a pan of water to the boil, add rice, cover and simmer for 20 minutes.

Add the peas to the pan in the last 5 minutes of cooking time.

Drain and cover the rice and return to the stove for 5 minutes.

When chicken is cooked through, serve on a bed of rice and peas and squeeze fresh lime juice over the top.

Enjoy.

Nutrition:
Calories: 220
Fat: 8g
Carbohydrates: 24g
Phosphorus: 172mg
Potassium: 293mg
Sodium: 210mg
Protein: 15g

Cajun Chicken and Shrimp Fiesta

Preparation Time: 10 minutes
Cooking Time: 40 minutes
Servings: 4
Ingredients:
1 tsp. cayenne pepper

1 tsp. paprika

1 tsp. dried oregano

1 tsp. dried thyme

1 tbsp. extra virgin olive oil

2 3oz skinless chicken breasts, chopped

1 white onion, chopped

1 garlic clove, crushed

8 fresh or frozen large shrimp

1 red bell pepper, chopped

3/4 cup white rice

1 cup water

Directions:
Mix the spices and herbs in a bowl to form your Cajun spice blend.

Grab a large pan and heat the olive oil on a medium to high heat.

Add the chicken and brown for around 4-5 minutes.

Remove chicken and place to one side.

Add the onion to the pan and fry until soft.

Now add the garlic, shrimp, Cajun seasoning and red pepper to the pan and cook for around 5 minutes or until prawns turn opaque.

Add the rice along with the chicken and water to the pan.

Cover the pan and simmer for around 25 minutes or until the rice is soft and the chicken is cooked through.

Serve hot!

Nutrition:
Calories: 186
Fat: 8g
Carbohydrates: 17g
Phosphorus: 160mg
Potassium: 315mg
Sodium: 310mg
Protein: 17g

Homemade Turkey Burgers

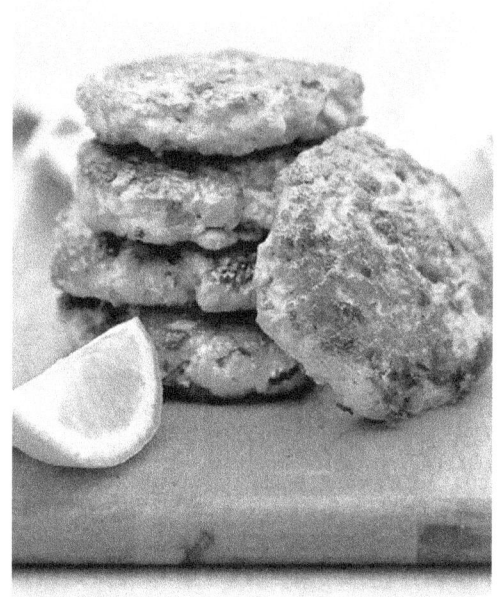

Preparation Time: 15 minutes
Cooking Time: 35 minutes
Servings: 2
Ingredients:
1/2 white onion, finely diced
1 celery stalk, finely diced
1/2 red bell pepper, finely diced
2 tbsp. olive oil
Pinch of black pepper to taste
1 tsp. dill
1 tsp. cilantro
1 tsp. dry mustard
3 oz lean ground turkey meat

2 hamburger rolls

1/2 cup arugula/baby spinach

Directions:

Pre-heat oven to 400°F/200 °C/Gas Mark 6.

Mix the vegetables, olive oil, pepper, herbs, and mustard in a medium bowl.

Add the meat to the vegetables and mix together until combined.

Use wet hands to 2 create burger patties.

Place the burgers on a lightly oiled baking tray and bake in the oven for 25-30 minutes or until meat is cooked through (use a knife in the center to check; the juices should run clear).

Serve in the hamburger roll and top with arugula/spinach and a helping of extra mustard as desired.

Nutrition:

Calories: 325

Fat: 20g

Carbohydrates: 23g

Phosphorus: 157mg

Potassium: 385mg

Sodium: 229mg

Protein: 15g

Spicy Chicken Fajitas

Preparation Time: 5 minutes
Cooking Time: 15 minutes
Servings: 6
Ingredients:
6 flour 4" tortillas
1/4 cup green pepper
1/4 cup red pepper
1/2 cup onion
2/3 cup green onions, sliced
2 tbsp. canola oil
6 oz. boneless chicken breasts
1/4 tsp. black pepper
1 tsp. chili powder
1/2 tsp. cumin
1/2 cup cilantro
2 tbsp. lemon juice

Directions:
Preheat oven to 300°F/150 °C/Gas Mark 2.

Wrap tortillas in foil and heat through in the oven for 10 minutes.

Meanwhile, chop the peppers, onions, and cilantro.

Cut chicken breasts into thin strips.

Place oil in a skillet over a medium heat.

Add the chicken, pepper, spices and lemon juice. Cook for 5-6 minutes.

Add the peppers and onion to the skillet and cook for a further 4 to 5 minutes or until chicken is completely cooked through.

Sprinkle the cilantro and squeeze the lemon juice over the chicken and fill the tortillas before wrapping.

Serve hot!

Nutrition:
Calories: 141
Fat: 7g
Carbohydrates: 10g
Phosphorus: 104mg
Potassium: 220mg
Sodium: 248mg
Protein: 10g

Ginger and Scallion Chicken Stir Fry

Preparation Time: 5 minutes
Cooking Time: 30 minutes
Servings: 4
Ingredients:
2 cup rice noodles, unsalted
1 tbsp. coconut oil
2x 3oz skinless chicken breasts
1 carrot, peeled and chopped
1/4 cup celery, chopped
1/2 cup chestnut mushrooms
1/2 cup scallions, chopped
1 tbsp. fresh ginger, grated
1 garlic clove, minced
1 lime

Directions:
Boil a pan of water on a high heat and add noodles. Cook for 10-15 minutes or according to package guidelines.

Meanwhile, heat oil in a wok on a high heat and add chopped chicken breasts.

Sauté for 15-20 minutes or until thoroughly cooked and place to one side.

Now add the carrot, celery and chestnut mushrooms to the same wok and cook for 10 minutes before adding scallions, ginger, garlic and cooked chicken back into the pan.

Stir through for a few minutes until piping hot throughout and add noodles to the wok after draining.

Serve with the juice of your lime squeezed over the top.

Nutrition:
Calories: 323
Fat: 6g
Carbohydrates: 52g
Phosphorus: 158mg
Potassium: 309mg
Sodium: 263g
Protein: 15g

Deep South Chicken Stew

Preparation Time: 10 minutes
Cooking Time: 40 minutes
Servings: 6
Ingredients:
3 cups cooked white
2 tbsp. canola oil
6 chicken drumsticks
1/2 cup onion, sliced
3/4 cup green bell pepper, sliced
2 tbsp. all-purpose flour
3 garlic cloves, minced
1/4 tsp. black pepper
1 dash red pepper
1/2 cup homemade chicken stock
1/2 cup water
Directions:
Prepare rice according to package directions (without salt).
Heat oil in a large pot over a medium to high heat.
Add chicken pieces to the skillet and brown on each side.
Add the onion and green pepper to the pan.
Sprinkle the flour over the ingredients in the skillet and stir to coat for a further 5 minutes.
Now add the garlic, black pepper, and red pepper.
Stir in the stock and water.
Cover pot and allow to simmer for approximately 30 minutes or until chicken is fully cooked and stock has thickened.
Serve over white rice.
Nutrition:
Calories: 249
Fat: 8g
Carbohydrates: 27g
Phosphorus: 164mg
Potassium: 260mg
Sodium: 73 mg
Protein: 15g

Chicken with Spiced Red Cabbage and Cranberry Sauce

Preparation Time: 2 minutes
Cooking Time: 30 minutes
Servings: 4
Ingredients:

1 red cabbage, sliced and soaked in warm water

1 tbsp. nutmeg

1 tbsp. extra virgin olive oil

1/4 red onion, finely sliced

6 oz. skinless, chicken breasts, sliced

1 cup cranberries

1 tbsp. apple vinegar

1 tsp. brown sugar

Directions:

Bring a pan of water to boiling point and add the sliced red cabbage with the nutmeg to the water.

Cover and simmer for 15-20 minutes.

Meanwhile, heat the oil in a skillet on a medium to high heat.

Add the onions and sauté for 5-6 minutes until soft.

Now add the chicken breasts for 10 minutes on each side.

In a separate small pan, add the cranberries with water to cover and the apple vinegar and brown sugar.

Bring to a boil and then turn down heat and simmer for 10 minutes or until cranberries are soft. Keep an eye on water levels and top up if necessary.

Once the cranberries are soft, blend in a food processor until smooth.

Drain the cabbage and season with black pepper.

Serve chicken breast on a bed of red cabbage and drizzle cranberry sauce over to taste.

Nutrition:
Calories: 213
Fat: 6g
Carbohydrates: 28g
Phosphorus: 121mg
Potassium: 298mg
Sodium: 235 mg
Protein: 14g

Aromatic Chicken and Eggplant Curry

Preparation Time: 10 minutes
Cooking Time: 35 minutes
Servings: 4
Ingredients:
1 tbsp. coconut oil
1/2 white onion, diced
1 tsp. garam masala
1 tsp. cumin
1 tsp. turmeric
1 clove garlic, minced
1/2 cup chopped tomatoes, no added salt or sugar
1 cup water
2x 2 oz. skinless chicken breasts, chopped
1 cup eggplant, soaked in warm water and cubed
2 cups white rice
2 tbsp. fresh cilantro, finely chopped

Directions:

Heat oil in a pan on a medium heat and add onions, stirring for 3-4 minutes until they begin to soften.

Add spices one by one and stir for 4-5 minutes, releasing the flavors.

Now add the garlic and stir.

Add the tomatoes and water to the pan and stir thoroughly.

Now add the chicken pieces and eggplant, cover and simmer for 25-30 minutes until chicken is completely cooked through.

Meanwhile prepare your rice by bringing a pan of water to the boil, before adding rice and covering to simmer for 20 minutes.

Drain and cover the rice and return to the stove for 5 minutes.

Serve individual rice portions and the chicken curry over the top.

Sprinkle with fresh cilantro to serve.

Nutrition:
Calories: 200
Fat: 5g
Carbohydrates: 27g
Phosphorus: 117mg
Potassium: 264mg
Sodium: 144mg
Protein: 11g

Italian Chicken

Preparation Time: 10 minutes
Cooking Time: 20 minutes
Servings: 4
Ingredients:
1 tsp. dried thyme
1 tsp. dried rosemary
1 tsp. dried basil
2x 3oz skinless chicken breasts
1 tbsp. olive oil
1 garlic clove, minced
1/2 lemon
1 tsp. black pepper
Directions:
Combine herbs in a bowl.
Place 1 chicken breast onto a chopping board, sprinkle with 1/2 herb mix and cover with plastic wrap; use a meat pounder or rolling pin to flatten the chicken breast.
Repeat for the remaining chicken breasts and herb mix.
Heat half the oil in a non-stick pan over a medium heat and add chicken breasts.
Cook for 8 minutes on each side until thoroughly cooked through.
Add garlic to the pan and stir for 2 minutes.
In a dressing bowl, whisk lemon juice, the rest of the olive oil and black pepper.
Drizzle the lemon dressing over the chicken breasts to serve with your favorite rice or couscous and greens.
Nutrition:
Calories: 104
Fat: 5g
Carbohydrates: 2g
Phosphorus: 101mg
Potassium: 188mg
Sodium: 208 mg
Protein: 13g

Orange & Ginger Chicken Noodles

Preparation Time: 5 minutes
Cooking Time: 20 minutes
Servings: 2
Ingredients:

1 cup rice/buckwheat noodles

2 tsp. coconut oil

3 oz. skinless chicken breast, chopped

1/2 cup scallions, chopped and soaked in warm water

1/4 cup bean sprouts, soaked in warm water

1 thumb sized piece of ginger, minced

1/2 orange, juiced

1 radish, soaked in warm water sliced to serve

Directions:

Cook the rice/noodles in a pan of boiling water for 10-12 minutes or according to package instructions.

Meanwhile, heat 1 tsp. oil in a skillet over a medium heat.

Sauté the chopped chicken breast for 10-15 minutes or until thoroughly cooked through.

Add the scallions and bean sprouts for the last 5 minutes and sauté.

In a separate bowl, mix together the ginger, 1 tsp. oil and orange juice.

Once chicken and noodles are cooked and drained, add all of the cooked ingredients along with the sliced radish to the dressing and toss through.

Serve warm or chilled.

Tip: layer a mason jar or sealable container so you can enjoy your delicious, healthy lunch on the go.

Tip: Use lime instead of orange if you have been advised not to include oranges in your diet - check with your doctor if unsure.

Nutrition:
Calories: 344
Fat: 7g
Carbohydrates: 54g
Phosphorus: 157mg
Potassium: 345mg
Sodium: 250mg
Protein: 15g

Lebanese Chicken Kebabs and Red Onion Salsa

Preparation Time: 15 minutes
Cooking Time: 25 minutes
Servings: 4
Ingredients:
2 tbsp. lemon juice
4 garlic cloves, minced
1 tbsp. thyme, finely chopped
1 tbsp. paprika
2 tsp. ground cumin
1 tsp. cayenne pepper
6oz skinless chicken breasts, cubed
4 metal kebab skewers
1 red onion, finely diced
1 red bell pepper, finely diced
1 tbsp. extra virgin olive oil
1 lime, juiced
1 tsp. black pepper
1 tbsp. fresh cilantro, finely chopped
Lemon wedges to garnish

Directions:
Whisk the lemon juice, garlic, thyme, paprika, cumin, and cayenne pepper in a bowl.

Skewer the chicken cubes using kebab sticks (metal).

Baste the chicken on each side with the marinade, covering for as long as possible in the fridge (the lemon juice will tenderize the meat which is great for anti-inflammation, one of the symptoms of kidney disease).

When ready to cook, preheat the oven to 400°F/200 °C/Gas Mark 6 and bake for 20-25 minutes or until chicken is thoroughly cooked through.

Prepare the salsa by mixing all salsa ingredients in a separate bowl.

Serve the chicken kebabs, garnished with the lemon wedges and the salsa on the side.

Nutrition:

Calories: 148

Fat: 6g

Carbohydrates: 11g

Phosphorus: 139mg

Potassium: 396mg

Sodium: 213 mg

Protein: 14g

Mediterranean Chicken and Zucchini Pasta

Preparation Time: 1 hour
Cooking Time: 30 minutes
Servings: 4
Ingredients:

2x 2 oz. skinless chicken breasts, sliced

2 tbsp. extra virgin olive oil

Juice of 1/2 lemon

1 clove garlic, crushed

1/2 tsp. dried oregano

Pinch of black pepper

3 zucchinis,

1 tsp. extra virgin olive oil

Directions:

Marinate the chicken slices in 1 tbsp. olive oil, lemon, garlic, oregano and pepper for at least 1 hour and up to overnight.

Pre-heat oven to 400°F/200°C/Gas Mark 6 when ready to cook.

Line a baking sheet with foil or parchment paper.

Layer the chicken strips on the baking tray and cook for 20-25 minutes or until cooked through.

Meanwhile, prepare your zucchini by slicing into thin spaghetti strips – use a mandolin or spiralizer and leave in a colander to drain for 10 minutes.

When chicken is cooked through, remove from oven and place to one side.

Boil a pan of water on a medium heat and add a pinch of black pepper.

Add your zucchini spaghetti to the water and boil for 2 minutes before immediately draining.

Plate and serve, layering the chicken on top and drizzling with 1 tsp. olive oil and a little black pepper.

Nutrition:
Calories: 144
Fat: 9g
Carbohydrates: 6g
Phosphorus: 119mg
Potassium: 371mg
Sodium: 140mg
Protein: 10g

Walnut and Basil Chicken Delight

Preparation Time: 10 minutes
Cooking Time: 35 minutes
Servings: 2
Ingredients:
2x 3oz skinless chicken or turkey 3oz skinless chicken breast
1/4 cup crushed walnuts
1/2 cup arugula
1 bunch of fresh basil
1/2 cup raw spinach
2 tbsp. extra virgin olive oil
1/4 cup brie (optional)
Directions:
Preheat oven to 350°f/170°c/Gas Mark 4.
Take the chicken breasts and use a meat pounder to 'thin' each breast into 1cm thick escalopes.
Reserve a handful of the nuts and arugula.
Add the rest of the ingredients and a little black pepper to a blender or pestle and mortar and blend until smooth (you can leave this a little chunky for a rustic feel if you wish).
Add a little water if the pesto needs thinning.
Coat the chicken in the pesto.
Bake the chicken in the oven for at least 30 minutes or until chicken is completely cooked through.
Top each chicken escalope with the remaining nuts and place under the broiler for 5 minutes for a crispy topping to complete.
Serve on a bed of arugula.
Nutrition:
Calories: 321
Fat: 29g
Carbohydrates: 3g
Phosphorus: 159mg
Potassium: 257mg
Sodium: 137mg
Protein: 15g

Chinese Chicken

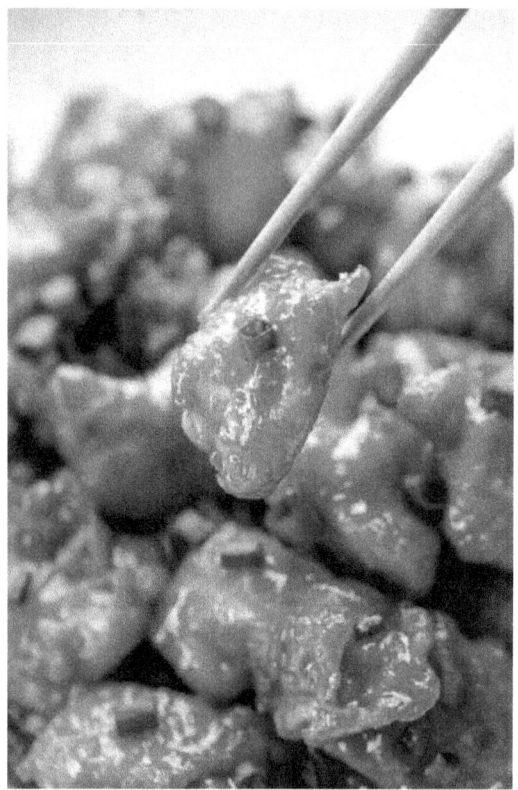

Preparation Time: 5 minutes
Cooking Time: 20 minutes
Servings: 6
Ingredients:
8 oz. lo mien noodles
2 tbsp. olive oil
6 oz. boneless, skinless, chicken breasts, sliced
1 cup onion, sliced
1-1/2 cups carrots, sliced
1 cup celery, sliced
1 cup mushrooms, sliced
1 tbsp. reduced-sodium soy sauce

Directions:

Bring a pan of water to the boil and cook noodles for 10-12 minutes or according to package directions.

Drain and place to one side.

Heat olive oil in a wok or skillet over a medium to high heat.

Add chicken and sauté for 10-15 minutes.

Ensure chicken has turned white on each side.

Now add onions, carrots, and celery.

Stir-fry gently for 5 minutes.

Add the mushrooms, soy sauce and drained noodles, stirring until heated through.

Ensure chicken is completely cooked through.

Nutrition:

Calories: 187

Fat: 6g

Carbohydrates: 22g

Phosphorus: 155mg

Potassium: 392mg

Sodium: 283 mg

Protein: 13g

Chicken and Mushroom Quesadillas

Preparation Time: 15 minutes
Cooking Time: 20 minutes
Servings: 12 to 16
Ingredients:

1/4 cup butter

2 1/2 tsps. chili powder

2 garlic cloves, minced

1 tsp. dried oregano

4 oz. fresh shiitake mushrooms, stemmed, sliced

4 oz. button mushrooms, sliced

1 1/2 cups shredded cooked chicken

2/3 cup finely chopped onion

1/3 cup chopped fresh cilantro

2 1/2 cups grated Monterey Jack cheese

Olive oil

16 5 1/2-inch-diameter corn tortillas

Directions:

In a big skillet, heat butter over medium-high heat until melted. Add oregano, garlic, and chili powder. Sauté for 1 minute until aromatic. Add button mushrooms and shiitake and sauté for 10 minutes until soft. Take away from heat. Stir in cilantro, onion, and chicken. Let cool for 10 minutes. Stir in cheese. Use pepper and salt to season (You can prepare this 8 hours in advance. Put a cover on and refrigerate).

Make the barbecue (medium heat). Lightly brush over one side of 8 tortillas with oil. On a big baking sheet, put the tortillas with the oiled side turning down. Divide among the tortillas with the chicken mixture, spreading until the thickness is even. Put the leftover 8 tortillas on top, press, and then brush oil over. Grill the quesadillas for 3 minutes each side until fully heated and golden brown. Slice into wedges.

Nutrition:

Calories: 223

Total Carbohydrate: 14 g

Cholesterol: 41 mg

Total Fat: 14 g

Fiber: 2 g

Protein: 12 g

Sodium: 181 mg

Saturated Fat: 7 g

Chapter 6: Meat Recipes

Spiced Lamb Burgers

Preparation Time: 10 minutes
Cooking Time: 20 minutes
Servings: 2
Ingredients:
1 tbsp. extra virgin olive oil
1 tsp. cumin
½ finely diced red onion
1 minced garlic clove
1 tsp. harissa spices
1 cup arugula
1 juiced lemon
6 oz. lean ground lamb
1 tbsp. parsley
½ cup low-fat plain yogurt
Directions:
Preheat the broiler on a medium to high heat.
Mix together the ground lamb, red onion, parsley, Harissa spices and olive oil until combined.
Shape 1-inch thick patties using wet hands.
Add the patties to a baking tray and place under the broiler for 7-8 minutes on each side or until thoroughly cooked through.
Mix the yogurt, lemon juice and cumin and serve over the lamb burgers with a side salad of arugula.
Nutrition:
Calories 306
Fat 20g
Carbs 10g
Phosphorus 269mg
Potassium (K) 492mg
Sodium (Na) 86mg
Protein 23g

Pork Loins with Leeks

Preparation Time: 10 minutes
Cooking Time: 35 minutes
Servings: 2
Ingredients:

1 sliced leek

1 tbsp. mustard seeds

6 oz. Pork tenderloin

1 tbsp. cumin seeds

1 tbsp. dry mustard

1 tbsp. extra virgin oil

Directions:

Preheat the broiler to medium high heat.

In a dry skillet heat mustard and cumin seeds until they start to pop (3-5 minutes).

Grind seeds using a pestle and mortar or blender and then mix in the dry mustard.

Coat the pork on both sides with the mustard blend and add to a baking tray to broil for 25-30 minutes or until cooked through. Turn once halfway through.

Remove and place to one side.

Heat the oil in a pan on medium heat and add the leeks for 5-6 minutes or until soft.

Serve the pork tenderloin on a bed of leeks and enjoy!

Nutrition:

Calories 139

Fat 5g

Carbs 2g

Phosphorus 278mg

Potassium (K) 45mg

Sodium (Na) 47mg

Protein 18g

Chinese Beef Wraps

Preparation Time: 10 minutes
Cooking Time: 30 minutes
Servings: 2
Ingredients:
2 iceberg lettuce leaves
½ diced cucumber
1 tsp. canola oil
5 oz. lean ground beef
1 tsp. ground ginger
1 tbsp. chili flakes
1 minced garlic clove
1 tbsp. rice wine vinegar

Directions:
Mix the ground meat with the garlic, rice wine vinegar, chili flakes and ginger in a bowl.

Heat oil in a skillet over medium heat.

Add the beef to the pan and cook for 20-25 minutes or until cooked through.

Serve beef mixture with diced cucumber in each lettuce wrap and fold.

Nutrition:
Calories 156
Fat 2g
Carbs 4 g
Phosphorus 1 mg
Potassium (K) 78mg
Sodium (Na) 54mg
Protein 14g

Grilled Skirt Steak

Preparation Time: 15 minutes
Cooking Time: 8-9 minutes
Servings: 4
Ingredients:
2 teaspoons fresh ginger herb, grated finely
2 teaspoons fresh lime zest, grated finely
¼ cup coconut sugar
2 teaspoons fish sauce
2 tablespoons fresh lime juice
½ cup coconut milk
1-pound beef skirt steak, trimmed and cut into 4-inch slices lengthwise
Salt, to taste

Directions:
In a sizable sealable bag, mix together all ingredients except steak and salt.
Add steak and coat with marinade generously.
Seal the bag and refrigerate to marinate for about 4-12 hours.
Preheat the grill to high heat. Grease the grill grate.
Remove steak from refrigerator and discard the marinade.
With a paper towel, dry the steak and sprinkle with salt evenly.
Cook the steak for approximately 3½ minutes.
Flip the medial side and cook for around 2½-5 minutes or till desired doneness.
Remove from grill pan and keep side for approximately 5 minutes before slicing.
With a clear, crisp knife cut into desired slices and serve.

Nutrition:
Calories: 465
Fat: 10g
Carbohydrates: 22g
Fiber: 0g
Protein: 37g

Spicy Lamb Curry

Preparation Time: 15 minutes
Cooking Time: 2 hours 15 minutes
Servings: 6-8

Ingredients:

4 teaspoons ground coriander
4 teaspoons ground coriander
4 teaspoons ground cumin
¾ teaspoon ground ginger
2 teaspoons ground cinnamon
½ teaspoon ground cloves
½ teaspoon ground cardamom
2 tablespoons sweet paprika
½ tablespoon cayenne pepper
2 teaspoons chili powder
2 teaspoons salt
1 tablespoon coconut oil
2 pounds boneless lamb, trimmed and cubed into 1-inch size
Salt and freshly ground black pepper, to taste
2 cups onions, chopped
1¼ cups water
1 cup coconut milk

Directions:

For spice mixture in a bowl, mix together all spices. Keep aside.

Season the lamb with salt and black pepper.

In a large Dutch oven, heat oil on medium-high heat.

Add lamb and stir fry for around 5 minutes.

Add onion and cook approximately 4-5 minutes.

Stir in spice mixture and cook approximately 1 minute.

Add water and coconut milk and provide to some boil on high heat.

Reduce the heat to low and simmer, covered for approximately 1-120 minutes or till desired doneness of lamb.

Uncover and simmer for approximately 3-4 minutes.

Serve hot.

Nutrition:

Calories: 466

Fat: 10g

Carbohydrates: 23g

Fiber: 9g

Protein: 36g

Lamb with Prunes

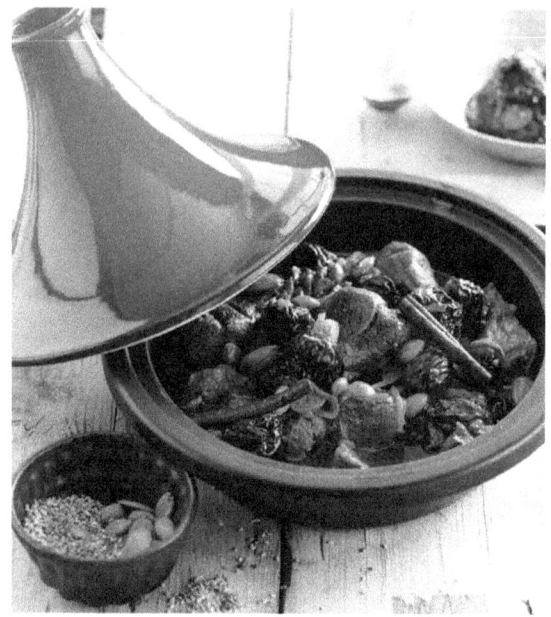

Preparation Time: 15 minutes
Cooking Time: 2 hours and 40 minutes
Servings: 4-6
Ingredients:
3 tablespoons coconut oil

2 onions, chopped finely

1 (1-inch) piece fresh ginger, minced

3 garlic cloves, minced

½ teaspoon ground turmeric

2 ½ pound lamb shoulder, trimmed and cubed into 3-inch size

Salt and freshly ground black pepper, to taste

½ teaspoon saffron threads, crumbled

1 cinnamon stick

3 cups water

1 cup runes, pitted and halved

Directions:

In a big pan, melt coconut oil on medium heat.

Add onions, ginger, garlic cloves and turmeric and sauté for about 3-5 minutes.

Sprinkle the lamb with salt and black pepper evenly.

In the pan, add lamb and saffron threads and cook for approximately 4-5 minutes.

Add cinnamon stick and water and produce to some boil on high heat.

Reduce the temperature to low and simmer, covered for around 1½-120 minutes or till desired doneness of lamb.

Stir in prunes and simmer for approximately 20-a half-hour.

Remove cinnamon stick and serve hot.

Nutrition:

Calories: 393

Fat: 12g

Carbohydrates: 10g

Fiber: 4g

Protein: 36g

Roast Beef

Preparation Time: 25 minutes
Cooking Time: 55 minutes
Servings: 3
Ingredients:
Quality rump or sirloin tip roast
Direction:
Place in roasting pan o n a shallow rack
Season with pepper and herbs
Insert meat thermometer in the center or thickest part of the roast
Roast to the desired degree of doneness
After removing from over for about 15 minutes let it chill
In the end the roast should be moister than well done.

Nutrition:
Calories 158
Protein 24 g
Fat 6 g
Carbs 0 g
Phosphorus 206 mg
Potassium (K) 328 mg
Sodium (Na) 55 mg

Beef Brochettes

Preparation Time: 20 minutes
Cooking Time: 1 hour
Servings: 1
Ingredients:
1 ½ cups pineapple chunks
1 sliced large onion
2 lbs. thick steak
1 sliced medium bell pepper
1 bay leaf
¼ cup vegetable oil
½ cup lemon juice
2 crushed garlic cloves

Directions:
Cut beef cubes and place in a plastic bag
Combine marinade ingredients in small bowl
Mix and pour over beef cubes
Seal the bag and refrigerate for 3 to 5 hours
Divide Ingredients: onion, beef cube, green pepper, pineapple
Grill about 9 minutes each side

Nutrition:
Calories 304
Protein 35 g
Fat 15 g
Carbs 11 g
Phosphorus 264 mg
Potassium (K) 388 mg
Sodium (Na) 70 mg

Country Fried Steak

Preparation Time: 10 minutes
Cooking Time: 1 hour and 40 minutes
Servings: 3
Ingredients:
1 large onion

½ cup flour

3 tbsps. vegetable oil

¼ tsp. pepper

1½ lbs. round steak

½ tsp. paprika

Directions:
Trim excess fat from steak

Cut into small pieces

Combine flour, paprika and pepper and mix together

Preheat skillet with oil

Cook steak on both sides

When the color of steak is brown remove to a platter

Add water (150 ml) and stir around the skillet

Return browned steak to skillet, if necessary, add water again so that bottom side of steak does not stick

Nutrition:
Calories 248

Protein 30 g

Fat 10 g

Carbs 5 g

Phosphorus 190 mg

Potassium (K) 338 mg

Sodium (Na) 60 mg

Beef Pot Roast

Preparation Time: 20 minutes
Cooking Time: 1 hour
Servings: 3
Ingredients:
Round bone roast
2 - 4 lbs. chuck roast
Direction:
Trim off excess fat
Place a tablespoon of oil in a large skillet and heat to medium
Roll pot roast in flour and brown on all sides in a hot skillet
After the meat gets a brown color, reduce heat to low
Season with pepper and herbs and add ½ cup of water
Cook slowly for 1½ hours or until it looks ready
Nutrition:
Calories 157
Protein 24 g
Fat 13 g
Carbs 0 g
Phosphorus 204 mg
Potassium (K) 328 mg
Sodium (Na) 50 mg

Homemade Burgers

Preparation Time: 10 minutes
Cooking Time: 20 minutes
Servings: 2
Ingredients:

4 oz. lean 100% ground beef

1 tsp. black pepper

1 garlic clove, minced

1 tsp. olive oil

1/4 cup onion, finely diced

1 tbsp. balsamic vinegar

1/2oz brie cheese, crumbled

1 tsp. mustard

Directions:

Season ground beef with pepper and then mix in minced garlic.

Form burger shapes with the ground beef using the palms of your hands.

Heat a skillet on a medium to high heat, and then add the oil.

Sauté the onions for 5-10 minutes until browned.

Then add the balsamic vinegar and sauté for another 5 minutes.

Remove and set aside.

Add the burgers to the pan and heat on the same heat for 5-6 minutes before flipping and heating for a further 5-6 minutes until cooked through.

Spread the mustard onto each burger.

Crumble the brie cheese over each burger and serve!

Try with a crunchy side salad!

Tip: If using fresh beef and not defrosted, prepare double the ingredients and freeze burgers in plastic wrap (after cooling) for up to 1 month.

Thoroughly defrost before heating through completely in the oven to serve.

Nutrition:

Calories: 178

Fat: 10g

Carbohydrates: 4g

Phosphorus: 147mg

Potassium: 272mg

Sodium: 273 mg

Protein: 16g

Slow-cooked Beef Brisket

Preparation Time: 10 minutes
Cooking Time: 3 hours and 30 minutes
Servings: 6
Ingredients:

10 oz. chuck roast

1 onion, sliced

1 cup carrots, peeled and sliced

1 tbsp. mustard

1 tbsp. thyme (fresh or dried)

1 tbsp. rosemary (fresh or dried)

2 garlic cloves

2 tbsp. extra virgin olive oil

1 tsp. black pepper

1 cup homemade chicken stock (p.52)

1 cup water

Directions:

Preheat oven to 300°f/150°c/Gas Mark 2.

Trim any fat from the beef and soak vegetables in warm water.

Make a paste by mixing together the mustard, thyme, rosemary, and garlic, before mixing in the oil and pepper.

Combine this mix with the stock.

Pour the mixture over the beef into an oven proof baking dish.

Place the vegetables onto the bottom of the baking dish with the beef.

Cover and roast for 3 hours, or until tender.

Uncover the dish and continue to cook for 30 minutes in the oven.

Serve hot!

Nutrition:
Calories: 151
Fat: 7g
Carbohydrates: 7g
Phosphorus: 144mg
Potassium: 344mg
Sodium: 279mg
Protein: 15g

Apricot and Lamb Tagine

Preparation Time: 10 minutes
Cooking Time: 1 hour and 30 minutes
Servings: 3
Ingredients:
1 tbsp. of extra virgin olive oil
2 lean lamb fillets, cubed
1/2 onion, diced
1 tsp. cumin
1 tsp. turmeric
1 tsp. curry powder
1 cup of homemade chicken stock (p.52) or water
1 tsp. dried rosemary
1/2 cup canned apricots, juices drained and apricots rinsed
1 tsp. of chopped parsley

Directions:
Heat the olive oil in a large oven-proof pot over a medium to high heat on the stove.

Add the lamb to the pot and cook for 5 minutes until browned.

Remove lamb and place to one side.

Add the chopped onion to the pot and sauté for 5 minutes until starting to soften.

Sprinkle the cumin, turmeric and curry powder over the onions and continue to stir for 4-5 minutes.

Now add the lamb back into the pot with the chicken stock and rosemary.

Then cover the pot and leave to simmer on a low heat for 1-1.5 hours until the lamb is tender and fully cooked through.

Add the apricots 15 minutes before the end of the cooking time.

Plate up and serve with the chopped parsley to garnish.

Tip: Follow instructions 1-5 and then complete the remaining steps in a slow cooker/Dutch oven and leave on a medium heat overnight.

Nutrition:

Calories: 194

Fat: 9g

Carbohydrates: 13g

Phosphorus: 140mg

Potassium: 372mg

Sodium: 197mg

Protein: 15g

Lemongrass and Coconut Beef Curry

Preparation Time: 10 minutes
Cooking Time: 45 minutes
Servings: 5
Ingredients:
1 tbsp. coconut oil
2 garlic cloves, minced
6 oz. 100% grass-fed sirloin, sliced into strips and fat trimmed
1 tsp. of fresh ginger, grated
1 tsp. curry powder
1 stick of lemongrass, very finely diced
1/4 cup of homemade chicken stock (p.52)
1 cup of tender-stem or sprouting broccoli
1/2 white onion, chopped
1/2 cup low fat coconut milk
1 stem of green onion, sliced
1 1/2 cups cooked brown rice/white rice (check what your dietitian recommends)

Directions:
Heat the coconut oil and garlic in a large pan over a medium to high heat for 2 minutes.

Add the beef slices to the pan and brown each side for 2 minutes.

Once browned, remove beef from the pan and place to one side.

Mix the ginger, curry powder, lemongrass and ¼ of the homemade chicken stock in a separate bowl.

Pour the stock mix, along with the broccoli into the pan.

Add the beef back into the pan along with the chopped onions.

Add the last of the stock and coconut milk over the beef and simmer for 30-40 minutes or until piping hot and the beef is soft.

Serve piping hot with the green onion scattered over the top and rice on the side.

Tip: Check with your doctor or dietitian as to whether you can still have coconut milk. Alternatively use a non-dairy milk such as almond.

Nutrition:

Calories: 239

Fat: 11g

Carbohydrates: 26g

Phosphorus: 179mg

Potassium: 364mg

Sodium: 42mg

Protein: 11g

Chili Crispy Beef Noodles

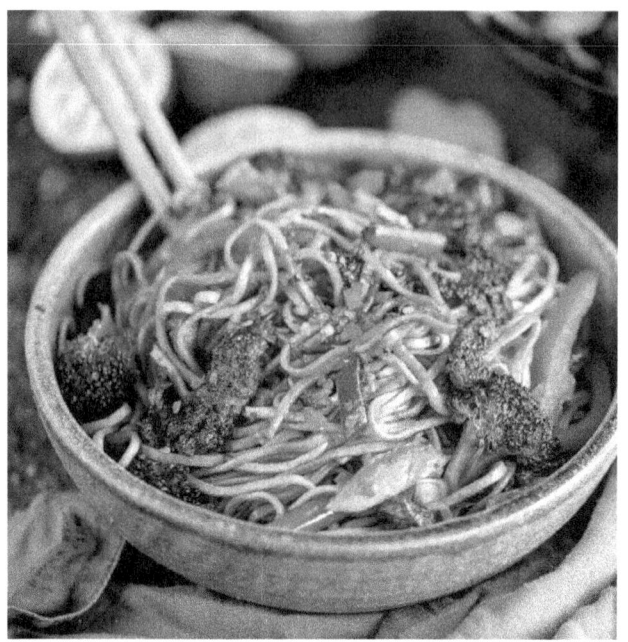

Preparation Time: 10 minutes
Cooking Time: 10-12 hours
Servings: 4
Ingredients:
1/2 small white onion
1 garlic clove, minced
2 tbsp. fresh parsley
8 oz. chuck roast, boneless & fat trimmed
5 cups water
1 bay leaf
1 tsp. black pepper
8 oz. rice noodles
2 tbsp. olive oil
1 tbsp. chili flakes
1 garlic clove, minced

1 stem green onion, finely chopped

1 lime

Directions:

Add all of the ingredients for the beef (up to and including black pepper) to a crock pot or slow cooker and cook on a medium heat for 10-12 hours or until very tender.

Remove the beef and shred the meat with a fork.

Cook noodles in a pot of boiling water for 10-15 minutes or according to package directions.

Whisk the olive oil, chili flakes, and garlic and add to a pan on a high heat.

Add the beef to the hot chili seasoning and cook on a high heat for 8-10 minutes or until crispy.

Scatter the green onions over the beef and stir.

Remove from the pan and portion over the noodles.

Squeeze the lime juice over the top to serve.

Nutrition:

Calories: 415

Fat: 17g

Carbohydrates: 51g

Phosphorus: 125mg

Potassium: 194mg

Sodium: 138mg

Protein: 14g

Harissa Lamb Burgers with Yogurt and Cumin Dip

Preparation Time: 10 minutes
Cooking Time: 20 minutes
Servings: 2
Ingredients:
5 oz. lean ground lamb
1/4 cup red onion, finely diced
1 tbsp. parsley
1 tsp. harissa spices
1 clove of garlic, minced
1 tbsp. extra virgin olive oil
1/2 cup arugula
1/4 lemon, juiced
1 tsp. cumin
1/2 cup non-dairy yogurt such as almond to serve (optional)

Directions:
Preheat the broiler on a medium to high heat.

Mix together the ground lamb, red onion, parsley, Harissa spices, garlic and olive oil until combined.

Shape 1 inch thick patties using wet hands.

Add the patties to a baking tray and place under the broiler for 7-8 minutes on each side or until thoroughly cooked through.

Plate up each burger and top with a helping of arugula.

Whisk the lemon juice and cumin and drizzle over the arugula topped burgers.

Nutrition:
Calories: 208
Fat: 16g
Carbohydrates: 4g
Phosphorus: 110mg
Potassium: 255mg
Sodium: 43mg
Protein: 12g

Mighty Meatloaf

Preparation Time: 10 minutes
Cooking Time: 30 minutes
Servings: 4
Ingredients:
1/2 white onion, diced
2 garlic cloves, minced
1 zucchini, grated
2 tbsp. extra virgin olive oil
1 tbsp. chopped fresh or dried parsley
7 oz ground lean pork
1/2 cup jarred red bell peppers, chopped
1/4 cup low fat coconut milk
2 large egg whites
1 tbsp. all-purpose flour
1 tsp. ground black pepper

Directions:
Preheat oven to 400°f/200°c/Gas Mark 6.
Soak vegetables in warm water for 10 minutes before draining.
Grease an oven-proof rectangular dish with 1 tbsp. olive oil.
Grab a skillet and heat 1 tbsp. oil on a medium heat.
Sauté the onion, garlic, zucchini with the parsley for five minutes, or until soft.
Place to one side to cool.
Add the pork, chopped peppers, coconut milk, egg whites, flour and black pepper to the vegetables and mix to combine.
Add the mixture to the oven dish and flatten the surface with a spoon.
Bake in the oven for 30 minutes or until thoroughly cooked through.
Remove and slice before serving with your choice of side dish.

Nutrition:
Calories: 248
Fat: 18g
Carbohydrates: 7g
Phosphorus: 145mg
Potassium: 403mg
Sodium: 258mg
Protein: 16g

Pulled Pork and Apple Buns

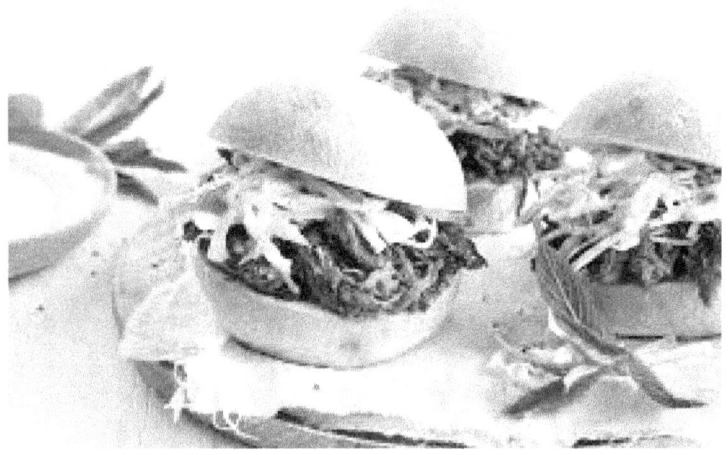

Preparation Time: 15 minutes
Cooking Time: 3-4 hours
Servings: 4
Ingredients:
1/2 onion, sliced
3 cloves garlic
8 oz. boneless pork shoulder roast
1 tbsp. extra virgin olive oil
1 cup water
1 tbsp. red wine vinegar
1 tsp. black pepper
2 cooking apples, peeled and chopped
3 tbsp. brown sugar
4 buns to serve

Directions:
Preheat oven to 350°f/180°c/Gas Mark 5.
Soak the onion and garlic in warm water.
Meanwhile, cut the pork into cubes.

In a skillet, cook the pork, onions, and garlic in the oil over a medium heat for 5 minutes.

Into a baking dish, add the water, red wine vinegar, and black pepper.

Cover and bake for 3-4 hours.

Remove the cover and continue to cook for 30 minutes.

Meanwhile, add the apples and brown sugar to a pot over a high heat and cover with water, allowing to simmer for 15-20 minutes or until apples are soft.

Remove pork from the oven and allow to cool before shredding the meat with a fork.

Whiz up the apples in a blender and serve in the buns with the pulled pork.

Enjoy!

Nutrition:

Calories: 270

Fat: 12g

Carbohydrates: 29g

Phosphorus: 124mg

Potassium: 277mg

Sodium: 168mg

Protein: 11g

Mustard and Leek Pork Tenderloin

Preparation Time: 10 minutes
Cooking Time: 35 minutes
Servings: 2
Ingredients:

1 tsp. mustard seeds

1 tsp. cumin seeds

1 tsp. dry mustard

6 oz. pork tenderloin

1 tsp. extra virgin olive oil

1 leek, sliced

Directions:

Preheat the broiler to a medium high heat.

In a dry skillet heat mustard and cumin seeds until they start to pop (3-5 minutes).

Grind seeds using a pestle and mortar or blender and then mix in the dry mustard.

Coat the pork on both sides with the mustard blend and add to a baking tray to broil for 25-30 minutes or until cooked through. Turn once halfway through.

Remove and place to one side.

Heat the oil in a pan on a medium heat and add the leeks for 5-6 minutes or until soft.

Slice and serve the pork tenderloin on a bed of leeks and enjoy!

Nutrition:

Calories: 165

Fat: 9g

Carbohydrates: 7g

Phosphorus: 154mg

Potassium: 309mg

Sodium: 67mg

Protein: 14g

Malaysian Style Lamb Curry

Preparation Time: 10 minutes
Cooking Time: 1 hour
Servings: 4
Ingredients:
1 tsp. olive oil
1 onion, diced
6 oz. lean lamb steaks, cubed
1 cup almond or rice milk (unenriched)
1 tsp. curry powder
1 eggplant, roughly chopped
1 tbsp. cilantro

Directions:
Heat oil in a pot over a medium to high heat and sauté onions for 5 minutes or until soft.

Add the lamb for 5-10 minutes, turning to brown each side, before adding the milk and curry powder.

Bring to the boil, then turn down the heat and add the eggplant to the curry.

Cover and simmer for 45-50 minutes or until the lamb is soft.

Scatter with cilantro and serve with rice or bread of your choice.

Tip: You could transfer the curry to a slow cooker and leave overnight to free you up from the stove if you wish - just ensure the liquid fully covers the lamb.

Nutrition:
Calories: 166
Fat: 6g
Carbohydrates: 12g
Phosphorus: 133mg
Potassium: 329mg
Sodium: 230mg
Protein: 15g

Chapter 7: Soup and Stew Recipes

Yucatan Soup

Preparation Time: 10 minutes
Cooking Time: 20 minutes
Servings: 4
Ingredients:
½ cup onion, chopped
8 cloves garlic, chopped
2 Serrano chili peppers, chopped
1 medium tomato, chopped
1 ½ cups chicken breast, cooked, shredded
2 six-inch corn tortillas, sliced
Nonstick cooking spray
1 tablespoon olive oil
4 cups chicken broth
1 bay leaf
¼ cup lime juice
¼ cup cilantro, chopped
1 teaspoon black pepper
Directions:
Spread the corn tortillas in a baking sheet and bake them for 3 minutes at 400°F.
Place a suitably-sized saucepan over medium heat and add oil to heat.
Toss in chili peppers, garlic, and onion, then sauté until soft.
Stir in broth, tomatoes, bay leaf, and chicken.
Let this chicken soup cook for 10 minutes on a simmer.
Stir in cilantro, lime juice, and black pepper.
Garnish with baked corn tortillas.
Serve.

Nutrition:
Calories: 214
Protein: 20 g
Carbohydrates: 12 g
Fat: 10 g
Cholesterol: 32 mg
Sodium: 246 mg
Potassium: 355 mg
Phosphorus: 176 mg
Calcium: 47 mg
Fiber: 1.6 g

Zesty Taco Soup

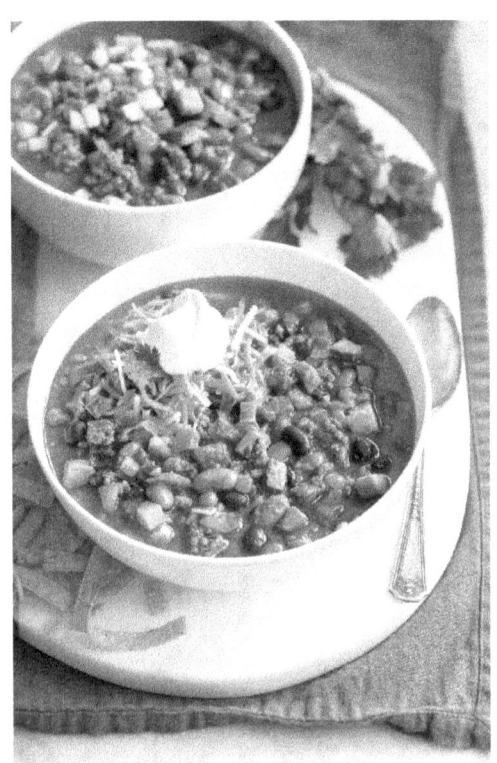

Preparation Time: 10 minutes
Cooking Time: 7 hours
Servings: 2
Ingredients:
1 ½ pounds boneless skinless chicken breast
15 ½ ounces canned dark red kidney beans
15 ½ ounces canned white corn
1 cup canned tomatoes, diced
½ cup onion
15 ½ ounces canned yellow hominy
½ cup green bell peppers
1 garlic clove

1 medium jalapeno

1 tablespoon package McCormick

2 cups chicken broth

Directions:

Add drained beans, hominy, corn, onion, garlic, jalapeno pepper, chicken, and green peppers to a Crockpot.

Cover the beans-corn mixture and cook for 1 hour on High temperature.

Reduce the heat to LOW and continue cooking for 6 hours.

Shred the slow-cooked chicken and return to the taco soup.

Serve warm.

Nutrition:

Calories: 190

Protein: 21 g

Carbohydrates: 19 g

Fat: 3 g

Cholesterol: 42 mg

Sodium: 421 mg

Potassium: 444 mg

Phosphorus: 210 mg

Calcium: 28 mg

Fiber: 4.3 g

Southwestern Posole

Preparation Time: 10 minutes
Cooking Time: 53 minutes
Servings: 4
Ingredients:
1 tablespoon olive oil
1 pound pork loin, diced
½ cup onion, chopped
1 garlic clove, chopped
28 ounces canned white hominy
4 ounces canned diced green chilis
4 cups chicken broth
¼ teaspoon black pepper

Directions:
Place a suitably-sized cooking pot over medium heat and add oil to heat.
Toss in pork pieces and sauté for 4 minutes.
Stir in garlic and onion, then stir for 4 minutes, or until onion is soft.
Add the remaining ingredients, then cover the pork soup.
Cook for 45 minutes, or until the pork is tender.
Serve warm.

Nutrition:
Calories: 286
Protein: 26 g
Carbohydrates: 15 g
Fat: 13 g
Cholesterol: 63 mg
Sodium: 399 mg
Potassium: 346 mg
Phosphorus: 182 mg
Calcium: 31 mg
Fiber: 3.4 g

Spring Vegetable Soup

Preparation Time: 10 minutes
Cooking Time: 45 minutes
Servings: 4
Ingredients:
1 cup fresh green beans, chopped
¾ cup celery, chopped
½ cup onion, chopped
½ cup carrots, chopped
½ cup mushrooms, chopped
½ cup frozen corn
1 medium Roma tomato, chopped
2 tablespoons olive oil
½ cup frozen corn
4 cups vegetable broth
1 teaspoon dried oregano leaves
1 teaspoon garlic powder
Directions:
Place a suitably-sized cooking pot over medium heat and add olive oil to heat.
Toss in onion and celery, then sauté until soft.
Stir in the corn and rest of the ingredients and cook the soup to boil.
Now reduce its heat to a simmer and cook for 45 minutes.
Serve warm.
Nutrition:
Calories: 114
Protein: 2 g
Carbohydrates: 13 g
Fat: 6 g
Cholesterol: 0 mg
Sodium: 262 mg
Potassium: 400 mg
Phosphorus: 108 mg
Calcium: 48 mg
Fiber: 3.4 g

Seafood Corn Chowder

Preparation Time: 10 minutes
Cooking Time: 12 minutes
Servings: 4
Ingredients:
1 tablespoon butter

1 cup onion, chopped

1/3 cup celery, chopped

½ cup green bell pepper, chopped

½ cup red bell pepper, chopped

1 tablespoon white flour

14 ounces chicken broth

2 cups cream

6 ounces evaporated milk

10 ounces surimi imitation crab chunks

2 cups frozen corn kernels

½ teaspoon black pepper

½ teaspoon paprika

Directions:

Place a suitably-sized saucepan over medium heat and add butter to melt.

Toss in onion, green and red peppers, and celery, then sauté for 5 minutes.

Stir in flour and whisk well for 2 minutes.

Pour in chicken broth and stir until it boils.

Add evaporated milk, corn, surimi crab, paprika, black pepper, and creamer.

Cook for 5 minutes then serve warm.

Nutrition:
Calories: 173
Protein: 8 g
Carbohydrates: 22 g
Fat: 7 g
Cholesterol: 13 mg
Sodium: 160 mg
Potassium: 285 mg
Phosphorus: 181 mg
Calcium: 68 mg
Fiber: 1.5 g

Beef Sage Soup

Preparation Time: 10 minutes
Cooking Time: 20 minutes
Servings: 4
Ingredients:
½ pound ground beef
½ teaspoon ground sage
½ teaspoon black pepper
½ teaspoon dried basil
½ teaspoon garlic powder
4 slices bread, cubed
2 tablespoons olive oil
1 tablespoon herb seasoning blend
2 garlic cloves, minced
3 cups chicken broth
1 ½ cups water
4 tablespoons fresh parsley
2 tablespoons parmesan cheese, grated

Directions:
Preheat your oven to 375ºF.
Mix beef with sage, basil, black pepper, and garlic powder in a bowl, then set it aside.
Toss the bread cubes with olive oil in a baking sheet and bake them for 8 minutes.
Meanwhile, sauté the beef mixture in a greased cooking pot until it is browned.
Stir in garlic and sauté for 2 minutes, then add parsley, water, and broth.
Cover the beef soup and cook for 10 minutes on a simmer.
Garnish the soup with parmesan cheese and baked bread.
Serve warm.

Nutrition:
Calories: 335
Protein: 26 g
Carbohydrates: 15 g
Fat: 19 g
Cholesterol: 250 mg
Sodium: 374 mg
Potassium: 392 mg
Phosphorus: 268 mg
Calcium: 118 mg
Fiber: 0.9 g

Cabbage Borscht

Preparation Time: 10 minutes
Cooking Time: 1 hour and 30 minutes
Servings: 6
Ingredients:

2 pounds beef steaks

6 cups cold water

2 tablespoons olive oil

½ cup tomato sauce

1 medium cabbage, chopped

1 cup onion, diced

1 cup carrots, diced

1 cup turnips, peeled and diced

1 teaspoon pepper

6 tablespoons lemon juice

4 tablespoons sugar

Directions:

Start by placing steak in a large cooking pot and pour enough water to cover it.

Cover the beef pot and cook it on a simmer until it is tender, then shred it using a fork.

Add olive oil, onion, tomato sauce, carrots, turnips, and shredded steak to the cooking liquid in the pot.

Stir in black pepper, sugar, and lemon juice to season the soup.

Cover the cabbage soup and cook on low heat for 1 ½ hour.

Serve warm.

Nutrition:
Calories: 202
Protein: 19 g
Carbohydrates: 9 g
Fat: 10 g
Cholesterol: 60 mg
Sodium: 242 mg
Potassium: 388 mg
Phosphorus: 160 mg
Calcium: 46 mg
Fiber: 2.1 g

Ground Beef Soup

Preparation Time: 10 minutes
Cooking Time: 30 minutes
Servings: 4
Ingredients:
1 pound lean ground beef
½ cup onion, chopped
2 teaspoons lemon-pepper seasoning blend
1 cup beef broth
2 cups of water
1/3 cup white rice, uncooked
3 cups frozen mixed vegetables
1 tablespoon sour cream
Directions:
Spray a saucepan with cooking oil and place it over medium heat.
Toss in onion and ground beef, then sauté until brown.
Stir in broth and rest of the ingredients, then boil it.
Reduce heat to a simmer, then cover the soup to cook for 30 minutes.
Garnish with sour cream.
Enjoy.
Nutrition:
Calories: 222
Protein: 20 g
Carbohydrates: 19 g
Fat: 8 g
Cholesterol: 52 mg
Sodium: 170 mg
Potassium: 448 mg
Phosphorus: 210 mg
Calcium: 43 mg
Fiber: 4.3 g

Shrimp and Crab Gumbo

Preparation Time: 10 minutes
Cooking Time: 15 minutes
Servings: 4

Ingredients

1 cup bell pepper, chopped

1 ½ cups onion, chopped

1 garlic clove, chopped

¼ cup celery leaves, chopped

1 cup green onion tops

¼ cup fresh parsley, chopped

4 tablespoons canola oil

6 tablespoons all-purpose white flour

3 cups of water

4 cups chicken broth

8 ounces shrimp, uncooked

6 ounces crab meat

¼ teaspoon black pepper

1 teaspoon hot sauce

3 cups cooked rice

Directions:

Prepare the roux in a suitably-sized pan by heating oil in it.

Stir in flour and sauté until it changes its color.

Pour in 1 cup water, then add onion, garlic, celery leaves, and bell pepper.

Cover the roux mixture and cook on low heat until the veggies turn soft.

Add 2 cups water and 4 cups broth, then mix again.

Continue cooking it for 5 minutes then add crab meat and shrimp.

Cook for 10 minutes then and parsley and green onion.

Continue cooking for 5 minutes then garnish with black pepper and hot sauce.

Serve warm with rice.

Nutrition:

Calories: 327

Protein: 22 g

Carbohydrates: 33 g

Fat: 11 g

Cholesterol: 86 mg

Sodium: 328 mg

Potassium: 368 mg

Phosphorus: 221 mg

Calcium: 79 mg

Fiber: 1.4 g

Tangy Turkey Soup

Preparation Time: 10 minutes
Cooking Time: 68 minutes
Servings: 4
Ingredients:

1 cup carrots, chopped

1 cup celery, chopped

1 cup green bell pepper, chopped

1 cup yellow onion, chopped

½ cup fresh tomato, chopped

½ cup fresh parsley, chopped

2 garlic cloves, chopped

1 cup mushrooms, sliced

2 cups zucchini, sliced

1 tablespoon olive oil

1 pound turkey breast, skinless, cubed

½ teaspoon black pepper

½ cup dry white wine

4 cups chicken broth

1 teaspoon dried thyme

1 bay leaf

¼ teaspoon crushed red pepper

3 cups white rice, cooked

3 tablespoons lemon juice

Directions:

Place a suitably-sized stockpot over medium heat and oil to heat.

Toss in turkey, and black pepper, then sauté for 10 minutes.

Stir in green bell pepper, onion, celery, and carrots, then sauté for 8 minutes.

Add garlic, tomato, and wine then cook for 2 minutes.

Stir in bay leaf, thyme, broth, and red pepper then cook for 30 minutes on a simmer.

Add zucchini, mushrooms, parsley, and rice to the soup then continue cooking for 15 minutes.

Serve warm with lemon juice on top.

Nutrition:

Calories: 214

Protein: 18 g

Carbohydrates: 22 g

Fat: 6 g

Cholesterol: 24 mg

Sodium: 128 mg

Potassium: 528 mg

Phosphorus: 197 mg

Calcium: 54 mg

Fiber: 2.4 g

Low Sodium Chicken Broth

Preparation Time: 5 minutes
Cooking Time: 4 hours
Servings: 10
Ingredients:

1 medium carrot, cut into 1-inch pieces

1 stalk celery, cut into 1-inch pieces

1 small onion, cut into 1-inch pieces

4lb skinless chicken leg quarters

6 sprigs fresh parsley

2 sprigs fresh thyme

1 bay leaf

1 garlic clove, minced

20 whole peppercorns

9 cup water

Directions:

Place all ingredients in a 6-quart slow cooker.

Cover and cook on HIGH for 4 hours.

Leave to cool and then strain well.

Use the cooked chicken for other dishes. The strained broth is flavorsome and the perfect base for countless dishes yet is virtually calorie and sodium-free. The broth can be refrigerated or frozen.

Nutrition:

Calories 34

Fat <1g

Carbs 3g

Protein 4g

Fiber 0g

Potassium 145mg

Sodium 39mg

Low Sodium Beef Broth

Preparation Time: 20 minutes
Cooking Time: 8 hours
Servings: 10
Ingredients:
3lb soup bones
1lb beef shank
4 large carrots, peeled and cut into 1-inch chunks
2 medium onions, peeled and chopped
2 tbsp. olive oil
2 bay leaves
5 garlic cloves, peeled and crushed
5 peppercorns
8 cup water
Directions:
Preheat oven to 400°F.
Place the bones, beef shank, and vegetables in a large roasting pan drizzled with the oil and roast for 2 hours until brown.
Place the beef, bones, and vegetables into a 5 or a 6-quart slow cooker along with the bay, garlic, and peppercorns.
Use 1 cup of water to scrape up the meat juices and add to the slow cooker with the remaining water.
Cover and cook on LOW for 8 hours.
Chill the broth overnight, then strain well to remove all the solidified fat.
The strained broth is flavorsome and the perfect base for countless dishes yet is virtually calorie and sodium-free. The broth can be refrigerated or frozen.
Nutrition:
Calories 20
Fat <1g
Carbs 0g
Protein 3g
Fiber 0g
Potassium 206mg
Sodium 20mg

Creamy Potato Soup

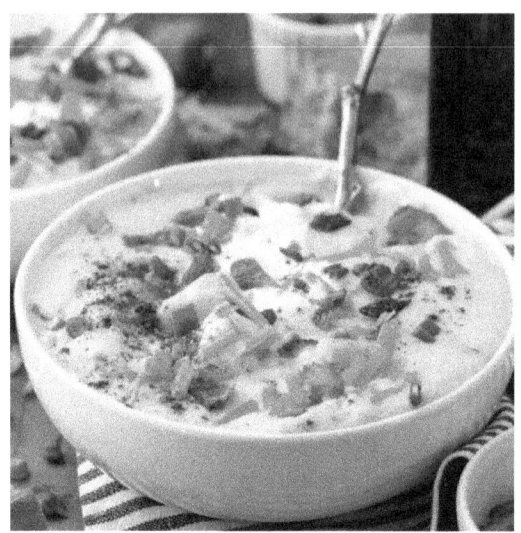

Preparation Time: 15 minutes
Cooking Time: 4 hours
Servings: 8
Ingredients:
Soup Ingredients
5 cup potatoes, peeled and diced
2 cup cauliflower, diced
2/3 cup celery, diced
1 cup onion, diced
6–8 cloves garlic, minced
4 cup sodium-free chicken broth (see recipe)
½ tsp. dried thyme
¼ tsp. dried cilantro
Roux Ingredients
1 tbsp. butter
¼ cup all-purpose flour
1 1/3 cup skim milk

¼ tsp. black pepper

½ tsp. low sodium salt

Directions:

Place all soup ingredients in a 5 to 6-quart slow cooker.

Cook on HIGH for 4 hours.

Puree the soup with a blender.

Make a roux by melting the butter and adding the flour in a small heavy-based pan.

Cook for 3 to 4 minutes.

Gradually add the milk until you have a thickened sauce.

Season the sauce, then stir into the soup and heat through before serving.

Nutrition:

Calories 396

Fat 18g

Cholesterol 61mg

Carbs 7g

Protein 20g

Fiber 2g

Potassium 1222mg

Sodium 420mg

Creamy Cauliflower & Butternut Squash Soup

Preparation Time: 5 minutes
Cooking Time: 2 hours
Servings: 6
Ingredients:
1 onion, diced
1-2 tsp. oil for sautéing
2-3 cloves garlic, minced
7 cup cauliflower florets
2 cup butternut squash, cubed
2 cup sodium-free vegetable or chicken broth (see recipe)
1 tsp. paprika
1 tsp. dried thyme
½ tsp. red pepper flakes
¼ tsp. low sodium salt
½ cup half and half

Directions:
Sauté onion and garlic in a heavy-based skillet.
Place in a 5 to 6-quart with all other ingredients except the half and half.
Cook on HIGH for 4 hours.
Puree the soup in a blender.
Stir in the half and half, heat through and serve.

Nutrition:
Calories 100
Fat 2g
Carbs 16g
Protein 3g
Fiber 6g
Potassium 553mg
Sodium 345mg

Crock Pot Turkey & Sweet Potato Chipotle Chili

Preparation Time: 15 minutes
Cooking Time: 4 hours
Servings: 8
Ingredients:
4 cup sweet potatoes, peeled and chopped
2– 2 ½ cup broth
1lb lean ground turkey
14 oz. diced low-sodium canned tomatoes
1 cup onion, chopped
2 –3 cup cauliflower, finely chopped
1 tsp. garlic, minced
2 chipotles, chopped
1 tsp. cumin
½ tsp. paprika
½ tsp. chili powder
¼ tsp. black pepper
½ tsp. low-sodium salt
½ cup bell peppers, chopped

Directions:
Par-cook the potatoes until tender and place in a 4 to 6-quart slow cooker.
Brown meat in a skillet, then add to slow cooker.
Add all remaining ingredients to slow cooker and mix well.
Cover and cook on HIGH for 3-4 hrs.
Check the seasoning and garnish with fresh cilantro and finely chopped jalapenos.

Nutrition:
Calories 311
Fat 12g
Carbs 21g
Protein 19g
Fiber 2g
Potassium 565mg
Sodium 211mg

Beef & Barley Stew

Preparation Time: 5 minutes
Cooking Time: 6-8 hours
Servings: 6
Ingredients:
1 cup pearl barley, uncooked
1lb lean beef stew meat, cut into 1-inch cubes
2 tbsp. all-purpose white flour
¼ tsp. black pepper
½ tsp. low-sodium salt
2 tbsp. canola oil
½ cup onion
1 large stalk celery, diced
1 garlic clove, minced
2 medium carrots, diced
2 bay leaves
2 quarts water
1 tsp. salt-free Mrs. Dash® onion herb seasoning

Directions:
Soak barley in 2 cups of water for 1 hour. Place in a 4-quart slow cooker.
Dust the meat in the black pepper and flour.
Heat the oil in a skillet and brown the meat. Add to the slow cooker.
Sauté the vegetables and garlic for a few minutes and add to the slow cooker.
Add the water and seasoning.
Cover and cook on LOW for 6-8 hours.

Nutrition:
Calories 246
Fat 8g
Carbs 21g
Protein 22g
Fiber 6g
Potassium 369mg
Sodium 150mg

Healthy Crockpot White Chicken Chili

Preparation Time: 30 minutes
Cooking Time: 6-8 hours
Servings: 8
Ingredients:
2-3 large boneless skinless chicken breasts
2 15.5oz cans of reduced-sodium great northern beans, drained and rinsed
1 15oz of sweet golden corn, drained well and rinsed
1 4.5oz can green chilies, chopped
4 cup chicken broth (see recipe)
1 medium sweet yellow onion, chopped
3 garlic cloves, minced
1 lime, juiced
1 tsp. cumin
½ tsp. onion powder
½ tsp. garlic powder
1 ½ tsp. chili powder
¼ tsp. cayenne pepper
1 tsp. black pepper
1 tsp. paprika

Directions:
Add chicken broth and squeeze the juice of one lime over the mixture.
Cook on LOW for 6 to 8 hours.
Before removing from the slow cooker, shred the chicken with forks.

Nutrition:
Calories 300
Fat 2g
Carbs 30g
Protein 32g
Fiber 6g
Potassium 549mg
Sodium 324mg

Green Chili Stew

Preparation Time: 20 minutes
Cooking Time: 10 hours
Servings: 6
Ingredients:
½ cup all-purpose flour
1 tbsp. garlic powder
1 tsp. black pepper
1lb lean boneless pork chops, cut into 1-inch cubes
1 tbsp. olive oil
1 8oz can of green chili peppers, drained well and chopped
1 garlic clove, minced
2 cup chicken broth (see recipe)
6 flour tortillas, burrito size
¾ cup iceberg lettuce, shredded
¼ cup cilantro, finely chopped
6 tbsp. sour cream

Directions:
Place the flour, garlic powder, and black pepper into a Ziploc bag.
Add the pork and coat well.
Heat the oil in a skillet and brown the pork.
Add the pork to a 4-quart slow cooker along with the broth, peppers, and garlic.
Cover and cook for 10 hours on LOW.
Place lettuce on a tortilla, top with stew and roll up burrito style.
Top with sour cream and cilantro.

Nutrition:
Calories 420
Fat 16g
Carbs 44g
Protein 25g
Fiber 3g
Potassium 454mg
Sodium 352mg

Turkey, Wild Rice, and Mushroom Soup

Preparation Time: 15 minutes
Cooking Time: 2-3 hours
Servings: 6
Ingredients:
½ cup onion, chopped
½ cup red bell pepper, chopped
½ cup carrots, chopped
2 garlic cloves, minced
2 cup cooked turkey, shredded
5 cup chicken broth (see recipe)
½ cup quick-cooking wild rice, uncooked
1 tbsp. olive oil
1 cup mushrooms, sliced
2 bay leaves
¼ tsp. Mrs. Dash® Original salt-free herb seasoning blend
1 tsp. dried thyme
½ tsp. low sodium salt
¼ tsp. black pepper

Directions:
Cook rice in a saucepan with 1-2 cups of broth. Set aside.

Heat oil in a skillet and sauté the onion, bell pepper, carrots, and garlic until soft. Add to a 4 to 6-quart slow cooker.

Add remaining ingredients to the slow cooker except for the rice and mushrooms.

Cover and cook for 2-3 hours on LOW.

Add the mushrooms and rice and cook for a further 15 minutes.

Remove the bay leaves and serve.

Nutrition:
Calories 210
Fat 2g
Carbs 15g
Protein 23g
Fiber 2g
Potassium 380mg
Sodium 115mg

Veggie Soup

Preparation Time: 20 minutes
Cooking Time: 6 hours
Servings: 6
Ingredients:
1 14oz no salt added diced tomatoes
1 large onion, diced
4 garlic cloves, minced
2 large carrots, diced
2 celery stalks, diced
1 medium parsnip, diced
1 large red bell pepper, diced
6 cup low sodium vegetable or chicken broth (see recipe)
3 cup cabbage, chopped
½ tsp. low sodium salt
½ tsp. black pepper
1 large sweet potato, peeled and diced

Directions:
Place all ingredients in a slow cooker.
Cook for 4-6 hours on HIGH.
Serve the soup chunky or puree if desired.

Nutrition:
Calories 135
Fat 1g
Carbs 30g
Protein 4g
Fiber 7g
Potassium 880mg
Sodium 250mg

Chapter 8: Vegetable Recipes

Thai Tofu Broth

Preparation Time: 5 minutes
Cooking Time: 15 minutes
Servings: 4
Ingredients:
1 cup rice noodles
½ sliced onion
6 oz. drained, pressed and cubed tofu
¼ cup sliced scallions
½ cup water
½ cup canned water chestnuts
½ cup rice milk
1 tbsp. lime juice
1 tbsp. coconut oil
½ finely sliced chili
1 cup snow peas

Directions:
Heat the oil in a wok on a high heat and then sauté the tofu until brown on each side.

Add the onion and sauté for 2-3 minutes.

Add the rice milk and water to the wok until bubbling.

Lower to medium heat and add the noodles, chili and water chestnuts.

Allow to simmer for 10-15 minutes and then add the sugar snap peas for 5 minutes.

Serve with a sprinkle of scallions.

Nutrition:
Calories 304
Protein 9 g
Carbs 38 g
Fat 13 g
Sodium (Na) 36 mg
Potassium (K) 114 mg
Phosphorus 101 mg

Delicious Vegetarian Lasagne

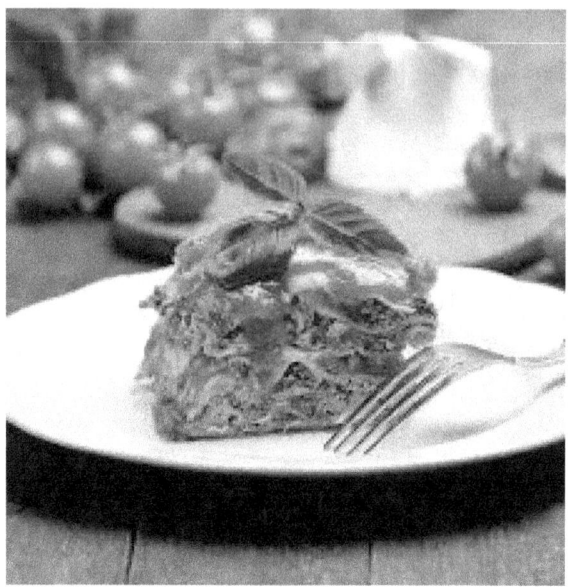

Preparation Time: 10 minutes
Cooking Time: 1 hour
Servings: 4
Ingredients:
1 tsp. basil
1 tbsp. olive oil
½ sliced red pepper
3 lasagna sheets
½ diced red onion
¼ tsp. black pepper
1 cup rice milk
1 minced garlic clove
1 cup sliced eggplant
½ sliced zucchini
½ pack soft tofu
1 tsp. oregano

Directions:

Preheat oven to 325°F/Gas Mark 3.

Slice zucchini, eggplant and pepper into vertical strips.

Add the rice milk and tofu to a food processor and blitz until smooth. Set aside.

Heat the oil in a skillet over medium heat and add the onions and garlic for 3-4 minutes or until soft.

Sprinkle in the herbs and pepper and allow to stir through for 5-6 minutes until hot.

Into a lasagne or suitable oven dish, layer 1 lasagna sheet, then 1/3 the eggplant, followed by 1/3 zucchini, then 1/3 pepper before pouring over 1/3 of tofu white sauce.

Repeat for the next 2 layers, finishing with the white sauce.

Add to the oven for 40-50 minutes or until veg is soft and can easily be sliced into servings.

Nutrition:

Calories 235

Protein 5 g

Carbs 10g

Fat 9 g

Sodium (Na) 35 mg

Potassium (K) 129 mg

Phosphorus 66 mg

Chili Tofu Noodles

Preparation Time: 5 minutes
Cooking Time: 15 minutes
Servings: 4
Ingredients:
½ diced red chili
2 cups rice noodles
½ juiced lime
6 oz. pressed and cubed silken firm tofu
1 tsp. grated fresh ginger
1 tbsp. coconut oil
1 cup green beans
1 minced garlic clove

Directions:
Steam the green beans for 10-12 minutes or according to package directions and drain.

Cook the noodles in a pot of boiling water for 10-15 minutes or according to package directions.

Meanwhile, heat a wok or skillet on a high heat and add coconut oil.

Now add the tofu, chili flakes, garlic and ginger and sauté for 5-10 minutes.

Drain the noodles and add to the wok along with the green beans and lime juice.

Toss to coat.

Serve hot!

Nutrition:
Calories 246
Protein 10 g
Carbs 28g
Fat 12 g
Sodium (Na) 25 mg
Potassium (K) 126 mg
Phosphorus 79 mg

Curried Cauliflower

Preparation Time: 5 minutes
Cooking Time: 20 minutes
Servings: 4
Ingredients:

1 tsp. turmeric

1 diced onion

1 tbsp. chopped fresh cilantro

1 tsp. cumin

½ diced chili

½ cup water

1 minced garlic clove

1 tbsp. coconut oil

1 tsp. garam masala

2 cups cauliflower florets

Directions:

Add the oil to a skillet on medium heat.

Sauté the onion and garlic for 5 minutes until soft.

Add the cumin, turmeric and garam masala and stir to release the aromas.

Now add the chili to the pan along with the cauliflower.

Stir to coat.

Pour in the water and reduce the heat to a simmer for 15 minutes.

Garnish with cilantro to serve.

Nutrition:

Calories 108, Protein 2 g

Carbs 11 g, Fat 7 g

Sodium (Na) 35 mg

Potassium (K) 328 mg

Phosphorus 39 mg

Chinese Tempeh Stir Fry

Preparation Time: 5 minutes
Cooking Time: 15 minutes
Servings: 2
Ingredients:
2 oz. sliced tempeh
1 cup cooked brown rice
1 minced garlic clove
½ cup green onions
1 tsp. minced fresh ginger
1 tbsp. coconut oil
½ cup corn

Directions:
Heat the oil in a skillet or wok on a high heat and add the garlic and ginger.

Sauté for 1 minute.

Now add the tempeh and cook for 5-6 minutes before adding the corn for a further 10 minutes.

Now add the green onions and serve over brown rice.

Nutrition:
Calories 304
Protein 10 g
Carbs 35 g
Fat 4 g
Sodium (Na) 91 mg
Potassium (K) 121 mg
Phosphorus 222 mg

Parsley Root Veg Stew

Preparation Time: 5 minutes
Cooking Time: 35-40 minutes
Servings: 4
Ingredients:
2 garlic cloves
2 cups white rice
1 tsp. ground cumin
1 diced onion
2 cups water
4 peeled and diced turnips
1 tsp. cayenne pepper
¼ cup chopped fresh parsley
½ tsp. ground cinnamon
2 tbsps. olive oil
1 tsp. ground ginger
2 peeled and diced carrots

Directions:

In a large pot, heat the oil on a medium high heat before sautéing the onion for 4-5 minutes until soft.

Add the turnips and cook for 10 minutes or until golden brown.

Add the garlic, cumin, ginger, cinnamon, and cayenne pepper, cooking for a further 3 minutes.

Add the carrots and stock to the pot and then bring to the boil.

Turn the heat down to medium heat, cover and simmer for 20 minutes.

Meanwhile add the rice to a pot of water and bring to the boil.

Turn down to simmer for 15 minutes.

Drain and place the lid on for 5 minutes to steam.

Garnish the root vegetable stew with parsley to serve alongside the rice.

Nutrition:
Calories 210
Protein 4 g
Carbs 32 g
Fat 7 g
Sodium (Na) 67 mg
Potassium (K) 181 mg
Phosphorus 105 mg

Mixed Pepper Paella

Preparation Time: 10 minutes
Cooking Time: 35-40 minutes
Servings: 2
Ingredients:
1 tbsp. extra virgin olive oil
½ chopped red onion
1 lemon
½ chopped yellow bell pepper
1 cup homemade chicken broth
½ chopped zucchini
1 tsp. dried oregano
½ chopped red bell pepper
1 tsp. dried parsley
1 cup brown rice
1 tsp. paprika

Directions:
Add the rice to a pot of cold water and cook for 15 minutes.
Drain the water, cover the pan and leave to one side.
Heat the oil in a skillet over medium-high heat.
Add the bell peppers, onion and zucchini, sautéing for 5 minutes.
To the pan, add the rice, herbs, spices and juice of the lemon along with the chicken broth.
Cover and turn the heat right down and allow to simmer for 15-20 minutes.
Serve hot.

Nutrition:
Calories 210
Protein 4 g
Carbs 33 g
Fat 7 g
Sodium (Na) 20 mg
Potassium (K) 33 mg
Phosphorus 156 mg

Cauliflower Rice & Runny Eggs

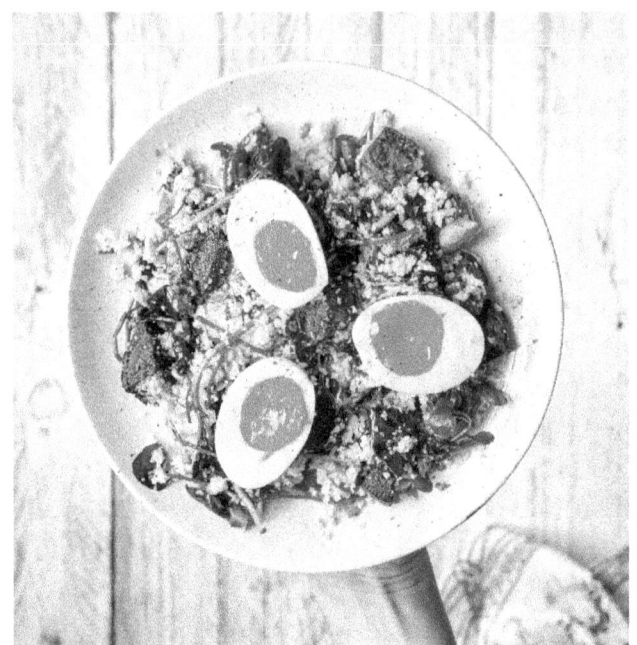

Preparation Time: 5 minutes
Cooking Time: 30 minutes
Servings: 4
Ingredients:
4 eggs
1 tbsp. extra virgin olive oil
1 tsp. black pepper
1 tbsp. chopped fresh chives
2 cups cauliflower
1 tbsp. curry powder
Directions:
Preheat the oven to 375°F/Gas Mark 5.
Soak the cauliflower in warm water in advance if possible. Grate or chop into rice-size pieces.

Bring the cauliflower to the boil in a pot of water and then turn down to simmer for 7 minutes.

Drain completely.

Place on a baking tray and sprinkle over curry powder and black pepper - toss to coat.

Bake in the oven for 20 minutes, stirring occasionally.

Meanwhile, boil a separate pan of water and add the eggs for 7 minutes.

Run under the cold tap, crack and peel the eggs before cutting in half.

Top the cauliflower with eggs and chopped chives.

Serve hot!

Nutrition:

Calories 120

Protein 7 g

Carbs 4 g

Fat 8 g

Sodium (Na) 175 mg

Potassium (K) 188 mg

Phosphorus 134 mg

Minted Zucchini Noodles

Preparation Time: 5 minutes
Cooking Time: 10 minutes
Servings: 2
Ingredients:

¼ deseeded and chopped red chili

2 tbsps. Extra virgin olive oil

½ juiced lemon

4 peeled and sliced zucchinis

½ cup chopped fresh mint

1 tsp. black pepper

½ cup arugula

Directions:

Whisk the mint, pepper, chili and olive oil to make a dressing.

Meanwhile, heat a pan of water on a high heat and bring to the boil.

Add the zucchini noodles and turn the heat down to simmer for 3-4 minutes.

Remove from the heat and place in a bowl of cold water immediately.

Toss the noodles in the dressing.

Mix the arugula with the lemon juice to serve on the top.

Enjoy!

Nutrition:

Calories 148

Protein 2 g

Carbs 4 g

Fat 13 g

Sodium (Na) 7 mg

Potassium (K) 422 mg

Phosphorus 256 mg

Chili Tempeh & Scallions

Preparation Time: 10 minutes
Cooking Time: 15 minutes
Servings: 2
Ingredients:
½ cup chopped scallions

1 juiced lime

1 tsp. soy sauce

2 oz. cubed tempeh

1 tbsp. grated ginger

1 tsp. coconut oil

½ deseeded and chopped red chili

Directions:

Mix the oil, soy sauce, chili flakes, lime juice and ginger together.

Marinate the tempeh in this for as long as possible.

Preheat the broiler to medium heat.

Add tempeh to a lined baking tray and broil for 10-15 minutes or until hot through.

Remove and sprinkle with scallions to serve.

Nutrition:

Calories 221

Protein 6 g

Carbs 8 g

Fat 10 g

Sodium (Na) 466 mg

Potassium (K) 189 mg

Phosphorus 99 mg

Cucumber-Carrot Salad

Preparation Time: 10 minutes
Cooking Time: 0 minutes
Servings: 2
Ingredients:

¼ cup rice vinegar

1 teaspoon sugar

½ teaspoon olive oil

1/8 teaspoon black pepper

½ cucumber, sliced

1 cup carrots, sliced

2 tablespoons green onion, sliced

2 tablespoons red bell pepper, sliced

½ teaspoon Italian seasoning blend

Directions:

Throw all the salad ingredients into a suitably-sized salad bowl.

Toss them well and refrigerate for 1 hour.

Serve.

Nutrition:

Calories: 25

Protein: 0 g

Carbohydrates: 6 g

Fat: 0 g

Cholesterol: 0 mg

Sodium: 22 mg

Potassium: 180 mg

Phosphorus: 22 mg

Calcium: 20 mg

Fiber: 1 g

Crunchy Couscous Salad

Preparation Time: 10 minutes
Cooking Time: 0 minutes
Servings: 4
Ingredients:
1 medium cucumber, sliced
½ cup red bell pepper, sliced
¼ cup sweet onion, sliced
2 tablespoon black olives, sliced
¼ cup parsley, chopped
½ cup couscous, cooked
2 tablespoons olive oil
2 tablespoons rice vinegar
2 tablespoons feta cheese crumbled
1 ½ teaspoon dried basil
¼ teaspoon black pepper

Directions:
Throw all the salad ingredients into a suitably-sized salad bowl.
Toss them well and refrigerate for 1 hour.
Serve.

Nutrition:
Calories: 121
Protein: 3 g
Carbohydrates: 14 g
Fat: 6 g
Cholesterol: 4 mg
Sodium: 167 mg
Potassium: 105 mg
Phosphorus: 51 mg
Calcium: 47 mg
Fiber: 1.4 g

Carrot and Jicama Salad

Preparation Time: 10 minutes
Cooking Time: 0 minutes
Servings: 2
Ingredients:
2 cup carrots, shredded
1 ½ cups jicama, shredded
1 tablespoon cilantro, chopped
2 tablespoons lime juice
1 tablespoon canola oil
1 tablespoon honey
Directions:
Throw all the salad ingredients into a suitably-sized salad bowl.
Toss them well and refrigerate for 1 hour.
Serve.
Nutrition:
Calories: 75
Protein: 1 g
Carbohydrates: 11 g
Fat: 3 g
Cholesterol: 0 mg
Sodium: 12 mg
Potassium: 130 mg
Phosphorus: 15 mg
Calcium: 12 mg
Fiber: 2.8 g

Green Beans with Bacon

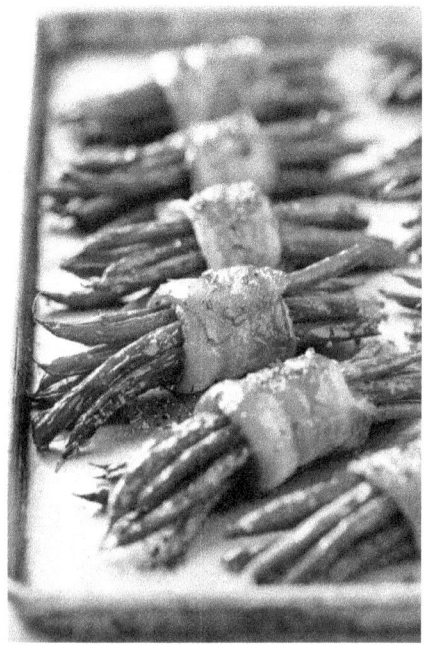

Preparation Time: 30 minutes
Cooking Time: 6-8 hours
Servings: 10
Ingredients:
12oz low-sodium bacon
29oz canned green beans
1 medium onion, chopped
½ cup maple syrup
¼ cup brown sugar

Directions:
Fry bacon and onion in a skillet and transfer to a 5 quart or larger slow cooker.

Add remaining ingredients and stir well.

Cover and cook on LOW for 6 to 8 hours.

Nutrition:
Calories 185
Fat 9g
Carbs 17g
Protein 12g
Fiber 1g
Potassium 125mg
Sodium 445mg

Coconut & Pecan Sweet Potatoes

Preparation Time: 20 minutes
Cooking Time: 4-5 hours
Servings: 16
Ingredients:

4lb sweet potatoes, peeled and diced

½ cup pecans, chopped

½ cup unsweetened flaked coconut

½ cup butter, melted

1/3 cup sugar

1/3 cup brown sugar

½ tsp. vanilla extract

¼ tsp. low sodium salt

Directions:

Place the sweet potatoes in a 5 quart or larger slow cooker.

Mix together the pecans, coconut, melted butter, both sugars, vanilla extract, and salt.

Toss the nut mixture with the sweet potatoes.

Cover and cook on LOW for 4 to 5 hours.

Nutrition:

Calories 307

Fat 16g

Carbs 42g

Protein 3g

Fiber 5g

Potassium 419mg

Sodium 50mg

Veggie Bolognese

Preparation Time: 20 minutes
Cooking Time: 8-10 hours
Servings: 32
Ingredients:
1 onion, diced
7 medium carrots, peeled & diced
2 green bell peppers, diced
3 small zucchinis, diced
2 cups mushrooms, roughly chopped
87oz canned crushed tomatoes
2 tbsp. dried basil
1 tbsp. dried oregano
1 tsp. dried rosemary
1 whole bay leaf, crumbled
3 garlic cloves, minced

Directions:
Place all ingredients into a 6-quart or larger slow cooker and mix well.
Cover and cook on LOW 8 to 10 hours.

Nutrition:
Calories 43
Fat <1g
Carbs 10g
Protein 2g
Fiber 3g
Potassium 411mg
Sodium 112mg

Bombay Potatoes

Preparation Time: 45 minutes
Cooking Time: 4-6 hours
Servings: 6
Ingredients:
3 tbsp. olive oil
2 tsp. mustard seeds
1 onion, peeled and diced
1 teaspoon Garam Masala Spice
1 tsp. ground ginger
1 ½ tsp. turmeric
½ tsp. ground cumin
½ tsp. chili powder
¼ tsp. red chili flakes
3lb potatoes, peeled and diced into ½ inch cubes
14.5oz canned low-sodium diced tomatoes or fresh tomatoes
1 tsp. low sodium salt
½ tsp. freshly ground black pepper
¼ cup fresh cilantro, finely chopped

Directions:
Cook the mustard seeds in a large skillet until they begin to pop.
Add the onions are spices and cook for a further 5 minutes.
Add the potatoes, tomatoes and onion mixture to a 6-quart slow cooker and cover.
Cook for 4 to 6 hours on LOW.

Nutrition:
Calories 280
Fat 8g
Carbs 10g
Protein 2g
Fiber 3g
Potassium 911mg
Sodium 78mg

Potato & Broccoli Gratin

Preparation Time: 20 minutes
Cooking Time: 3-4 hours
Servings: 6
Ingredients:
5 medium potatoes, sliced
2 cup broccoli florets, chopped
½ tsp. freshly ground black pepper
½ tsp. low sodium salt
¼ cup unsalted margarine
¼ cup all-purpose flour
1 medium onion, minced
1 garlic clove, minced
1 cup milk
1 cup low-sodium Cheddar cheese

Directions:
Arrange the potato slices and broccoli florets in a 4 to 6-quart slow cooker.

Melt the margarine in a saucepan and add the flour to make a roux.

Gradually whisk in the milk, then add the garlic, onion, and cheese.

Pour the sauce over potatoes and cover.

Cover and cook on HIGH for 3 to 4 hours.

Nutrition:
Calories 444
Fat 21g
Carbs 49g
Protein 2g
Fiber 7g
Potassium 1106mg
Sodium 378mg

Summer Squash with Bell Pepper and Pineapple

Preparation Time: 15 minutes
Cooking Time: 6-7 hours
Servings: 6
Ingredients:

1lb summer squash, peeled and cubed

1lb zucchini squash, peeled and cubed

½ cup green bell pepper, chopped

1 8oz can unsweetened crushed pineapple

1 tsp. ground cinnamon

1/3 cup brown sugar

1 tbsp. butter, cut into small pieces

Directions:

Mix all ingredients together and place in a 4 to 6-quart slow cooker.

Cover and cook on LOW for 6-7 hours or until squash is tender.

Serve immediately.

Nutrition:

Calories 113

Fat 2g

Carbs 24g

Protein 2g

Fiber 2g

Potassium 381mg

Sodium 7mg

Slow Cooker Eggplant Lasagna

Preparation Time: 20 minutes
Cooking Time: 2-3 hours
Servings: 8

Ingredients:

2 eggplants, peeled and sliced thin to resemble lasagna noodles

1 cup low-fat cottage cheese

1 ½ cup low-fat mozzarella cheese

1 egg

1 24oz jar sodium-free spaghetti sauce

1 tsp. low-sodium salt

1 bell pepper, diced

1 onion, diced

Directions:

Season the eggplants with salt and pepper, arrange on paper towels and allow excess moisture to drain away.

Mix the cottage cheese, mozzarella cheese, and egg in a bowl.

Pour ¼ of the tomato sauce in a 4 to 6-quart slow cooker.

Layer like lasagna with vegetables, cheese mix, and tomato sauce.

Cover and cook on LOW for 2 to 3 hours.

Nutrition:

Calories 221

Fat 10g

Carbs 19g

Protein 14g

Fiber 3g

Potassium 349mg

Sodium 802mg

Chapter 9: Egg and Animal Product Recipes

Mixed Pepper Mushroom Omelet

Preparation Time: 15 minutes
Cooking Time: 10 minutes
Servings: 2
Ingredients:

1/4 cup green onions, chopped

1/4 cup fresh mushrooms, sliced

1/4 cup green pepper, chopped

2 tablespoons butter, divided

5 eggs

1/4 teaspoon pepper

1/4 cup Cheddar cheese, shredded

1/4 cup Monterey Jack cheese, shredded

Directions:

Begin by sautéing all the vegetables with the butter in a pan until crispy.

Whisk the eggs and black pepper until foamy and fluffy.

Spread this egg mixture over the vegetables in the pan and cover with a lid.

Cook for about 2 minutes, then flip the omelet with a spatula.

Drizzle the cheese on top and cover the lid for 2 more minutes. Slice and serve.

Nutrition:

Calories 378

Total Fat 31.5g

Saturated Fat 16.4g

Cholesterol 467mg
Sodium 402mg
Carbohydrate 3.1g
Dietary Fiber 0.7g
Sugars 1.7g
Protein 21.6g
Calcium 280mg
Phosphorous 412mg
Potassium 262mg

Chicken Egg Rolls

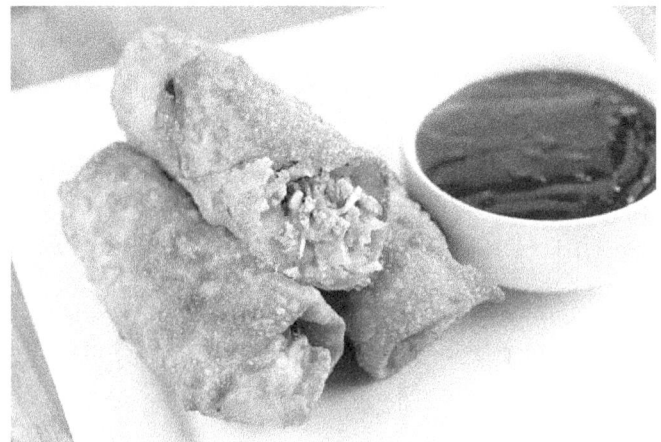

Preparation Time: 15 minutes
Cooking Time: 12 minutes
Servings: 14
Ingredients:
1 lb. cooked chicken, diced
1/2 lb. bean sprouts
1/2 lb. cabbage, shredded
1 cup onion, chopped
2 tablespoons olive oil
1 tablespoon low sodium soy sauce
1 garlic clove, minced
20 egg roll wrappers
Oil for frying

Directions:
Add everything to a suitable bowl except for the roll wrappers.

Mix these ingredients well to prepare the filling then marinate for 30 minutes.

Place the roll wrappers on the working surface and divide the prepared filling on them.

Fold the roll wrappers as per the package instructions and keep them aside.

Add oil to a deep wok and heat it to 350 degrees F.

Deep the egg rolls until golden brown on all sides.

Transfer the egg rolls to a plate lined with paper towel to absorb all the excess oil.

Serve warm.

Nutrition:

Calories 212

Total Fat 3.8g

Saturated Fat 0.7g

Cholesterol 29mg

Sodium 329mg

Carbohydrate 29g

Dietary Fiber 1.4g

Sugars 0.9g

Protein 14.9g

Calcium 37mg

Phosphorous 361 mg

Potassium 171mg

Mushroom Omelet

Preparation Time: 15 minutes
Cooking Time: 10 minutes
Servings: 2
Ingredients:
2 tablespoons and 1 teaspoon olive oil
1 shallot, minced
¼ lb. cremini mushrooms, rinsed
Black pepper to taste
1 garlic clove, minced
2 teaspoons parsley, minced
4 eggs
1 tablespoon chives, minced
2 teaspoons milk
3 tablespoons Gruyere cheese, grated

Directions:
Set a suitable non-stick skillet over moderate heat and add 1 teaspoon olive oil.
Add in the shallot and mushrooms, then sauté for 5 minutes until soft.
Toss in the garlic and sauté for 1 minute.
Now add the rest of the oil to the same skillet.
Mix the eggs with the chives, milk, and black pepper in a bowl and pour it into the skillet.
Cook the egg omelet for about 2 minutes per side until golden brown then transfers to the serving place.
Serve with Gruyere cheese and parsley on top.
Enjoy.

Nutrition:
Calories 271
Total Fat 23g
Saturated Fat 4.8g
Cholesterol 328mg

Sodium 208mg
Carbohydrate 4.8g
Dietary Fiber 0.5g
Sugars 2g
Protein 13g
Calcium 71mg
Phosphorous 227mg
Potassium 410mg

Onion Cheese Omelet

Preparation Time: 15 minutes
Cooking Time: 12 minutes
Servings: 2
Ingredients:
3 eggs
1/4 cup liquid creamer
1 tablespoon water
Black pepper to taste
1 tablespoon butter
3/4 cup onion, sliced
1 large apple, peeled, cored, and sliced
2 tablespoons Cheddar cheese, grated

Directions:
Switch your gas oven to 400 degrees F to preheat.
Whisk the eggs with the liquid creamer, water, and black pepper in a suitable bowl.
Stir ¼ of the butter into an oven safe skillet and sauté the onion and apple slices.
After 5 minutes, pour in the egg mixture over the onions.
Sprinkle Cheddar cheese over the egg and bake for approximately 12 minutes.
Slice the omelet and serve.

Nutrition:
Calories 254
Total Fat 15.1g
Saturated Fat 7.2g
Cholesterol 268mg
Sodium 184mg
Carbohydrate 20.7g
Dietary Fiber 3.6g
Sugars 14.6g
Protein 10.9g
Calcium 98mg
Phosphorous 334mg
Potassium 280mg

Eggs with Green Chilies

Preparation Time: 5 minutes
Cooking Time: 20 minutes
Servings: 2
Ingredients:
Egg whites – 1 cup
Whole eggs – 1
Cheddar cheese, shredded, low-sodium – .5 cup
All-purpose flour – 1 tablespoon
Black pepper, ground - .125 teaspoon
Parsley, dried – .5 teaspoon
Onion, diced - .25 cup
Garlic, minced – 2 cloves
Bell pepper, diced - .25 cup
Green chilled, canned, rinsed – 2 tablespoons

Directions:

Preheat your oven to a temperature of Fahrenheit three-hundred and fifty degrees and grease a regular-sized loaf pan for the egg casserole.

In a medium-sized bowl for the purpose of mixing whisk together the egg whites and whole egg until the two are completely combined. Whisk in the remaining ingredients.

Pour the prepared egg, vegetable, and cheese mixture into the greased loaf pan and then place it in the center of the oven, allowing it to cook until it has set and the eggs are cooked all the way through, about twenty to twenty-five minutes.

Nutrition:
Number of Calories in Individual **Servings:** 259
Protein Grams: 24
Phosphorus Milligrams: 343
Potassium Milligrams: 384
Sodium Milligrams: 238
Fat Grams: 13
Total Carbohydrates Grams: 8
Net Carbohydrates Grams: 8

Pepperoni Omelet

Preparation Time: 5 minutes
Cooking Time: 20 minutes
Servings: 2
Ingredients:
3 eggs
7 pepperoni slices
1 teaspoon coconut cream
Salt and freshly ground black pepper, to taste
1 tablespoon almond butter
Directions:
Take a bowl and whisk eggs with all the remaining ingredients
Then take a skillet and heat the butter
Pour one quarter of the egg mixture into your skillet
After that, cook for 2 minutes per side
Repeat to use the entire batter
Serve warm and enjoy!
Nutrition:
Calories: 141
Fat: 11.5g
Carbohydrates: 0.6g
Protein: 8.9g

Scrambled Turkey Eggs

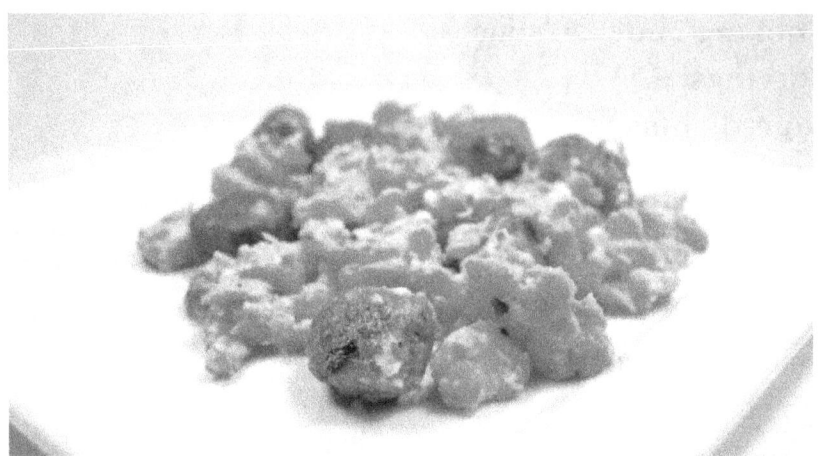

Preparation Time: 15 minutes
Cooking Time: 15 minutes
Servings: 2
Ingredients:
1 tablespoon coconut oil
1 medium red bell pepper, diced
½ medium yellow onion, diced
¼ teaspoon hot pepper sauce
3 large free-range eggs
¼ teaspoon black pepper, freshly ground
¼ teaspoon salt

Directions:
Set a pan to medium-high heat and add coconut oil, let it heat up
Add onions and Saute
Add turkey and red pepper
Cook until turkey is cooked
Take a bowl and beat eggs, stir in salt and pepper

Pour eggs in the pan with turkey and gently cook and scramble eggs

Top with hot sauce and enjoy!

Nutrition:

Calories: 435

Fat: 30g

Carbohydrates: 34g

Protein: 16g

Angel Eggs

Preparation Time: 30 minutes
Cooking Time: 0 minutes
Servings: 2
Ingredients:
4 eggs, hardboiled and peeled
1 tablespoon vanilla bean sweetener, sugar-free
2 tablespoons Keto-Friendly mayonnaise
1/8 teaspoon cinnamon
Directions:
Halve the boiled eggs and scoop out the yolk
Place in a bowl
Add egg whites on a plate
Add sweetener, cinnamon, mayo to the egg yolks and mash them well
Transfer the yolk mix to white halves
Serve and enjoy!
Nutrition:
Calories: 184
Fat: 15g
Carbohydrates: 1g
Protein: 12g

Denver Omelets

Preparation Time: 4 minutes
Cooking Time: 1 minutes
Servings: 1
Ingredients:
2 tablespoons almond butter
¼ cup onion, chopped
¼ cup green bell pepper, diced
¼ cup grape tomatoes halved
2 whole eggs
¼ cup ham, chopped
Directions:
Take a skillet and place it over medium heat
Add butter and wait until the butter melts
Add onion and bell pepper and sauté for a few minutes
Take a bowl and whip eggs
Add the remaining ingredients and stir
Add sautéed onion and pepper, stir
Microwave the egg mix for 1 minute
Serve hot!
Nutrition:
Calories: 605
Fat: 46g
Carbohydrates: 6g
Protein: 39g

Scrambled Eggs and Pesto

Preparation Time: 5 minutes
Cooking Time: 5 minutes
Servings: 2
Ingredients:
3 large whole eggs
1 tablespoon almond butter
1 tablespoon pesto
2 tablespoons creamed coconut milk
Salt and pepper as needed
Directions:
Take a bowl and crack open your egg
Season with a pinch of salt and pepper
Pour eggs into a pan
Add butter and introduce heat
Cook on low heat and gently add pesto
Once the egg is cooked and scrambled, remove from the heat
Spoon in coconut cream and mix well
Turn on the heat and cook on LOW until you have a creamy texture
Serve and enjoy!
Nutrition:
Calories: 467
Fat: 41g
Carbohydrates: 3g
Protein: 20g

Chapter 10: Dessert Recipes

Lemon Mousse

Preparation Time: 10 minutes + chilling time
Cooking Time: 10 minutes
Servings: 4
Ingredients:

1 cup coconut cream

8 ounces cream cheese, soft

¼ cup fresh lemon juice

3 pinches salt

1 teaspoon lemon liquid stevia

Directions:

Preheat your oven to 350 °F

Grease a ramekin with butter

Beat cream, cream cheese, fresh lemon juice, salt and lemon liquid stevia in a mixer

Pour batter into ramekin

Bake for 10 minutes, then transfer the mousse to a serving glass

Let it chill for 2 hours and serve

Enjoy!

Nutrition:

Calories: 395

Fat: 31g

Carbohydrates: 3g

Protein: 5g

Jalapeno Crisp

Preparation Time: 10 minutes
Cooking Time: 1 hour 15 minutes
Servings: 20
Ingredients:

1 cup sesame seeds

1 cup sunflower seeds

1 cup flaxseeds

½ cup hulled hemp seeds

3 tablespoons Psyllium husk

1 teaspoon salt

1 teaspoon baking powder

2 cups of water

Directions:

Pre-heat your oven to 350 °F

Take your blender and add seeds, baking powder, salt, and Psyllium husk

Blend well until a sand-like texture appears

Stir in water and mix until a batter forms

llow the batter to rest for 10 minutes until a dough-like thick mixture forms

Pour the dough onto a cookie sheet lined with parchment paper

Spread it evenly, making sure that it has a thickness of ¼ inch thick all around

Bake for 75 minutes in your oven

Remove and cut into 20 spices

Allow them to cool for 30 minutes and enjoy!

Nutrition:

Calories: 156

Fat: 13g

Carbohydrates: 2g

Protein: 5g

Raspberry Popsicle

Preparation Time: 2 hours
Cooking Time: 15 minutes
Servings: 4
Ingredients:
1 ½ cups raspberries
2 cups of water
Directions:
Take a pan and fill it up with water
Add raspberries
Place it over medium heat and bring to water to a boil
Reduce the heat and simmer for 15 minutes
Remove heat and pour the mix into Popsicle molds
Add a popsicle stick and let it chill for 2 hours
Serve and enjoy!
Nutrition:
Calories: 58
Fat: 0.4g
Carbohydrates: 0g
Protein: 1.4g

Easy Fudge

Preparation Time: 15 minutes + chill time
Cooking Time: 5 minutes
Servings: 25
Ingredients:

1 ¾ cups of coconut butter

1 cup pumpkin puree

1 teaspoon ground cinnamon

¼ teaspoon ground nutmeg

1 tablespoon coconut oil

Directions:

Take an 8x8 inch square baking pan and line it with aluminum foil

Take a spoon and scoop out the coconut butter into a heated pan and allow the butter to melt

Keep stirring well and remove from the heat once fully melted

Add spices and pumpkin and keep straining until you have a grain-like texture

Add coconut oil and keep stirring to incorporate everything

Scoop the mixture into your baking pan and evenly distribute it

Place wax paper on top of the mixture and press gently to straighten the top

Remove the paper and discard

Allow it to chill for 1-2 hours

Once chilled, take it out and slice it up into pieces

Enjoy!

Nutrition:

Calories: 120

Fat: 10g

Carbohydrates: 5g

Protein: 1.2g

Blueberry Muffins

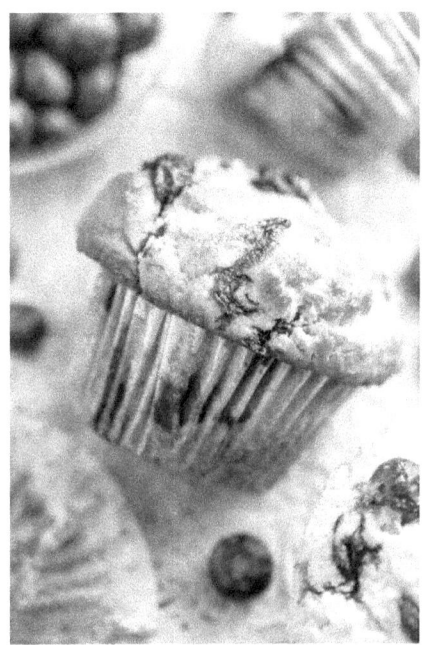

Preparation Time: 10 minutes
Cooking Time: 30 minutes
Servings: 4
Ingredients:
1 cup almond flour
Pinch of salt
1/8 teaspoon baking soda
1 whole egg
2 tablespoons coconut oil, melted
½ cup of coconut milk
¼ cup fresh blueberries
Directions:
Preheat your oven to 350 °F
Line a muffin tin with paper muffin cups

Add almond flour, salt, baking soda to a bowl and mix, keep it on the side

Take another bowl and add egg, coconut oil, coconut milk, and mix

Add mix to flour mix and gently combine until incorporated

Mix in blueberries and fill the cupcakes tins with batter

Bake for 20-25 minutes

Enjoy!

Nutrition:

Calories: 167

Fat: 15g

Carbohydrates: 2.1g

Protein: 5.2g

The Coconut Loaf

Preparation Time: 15 minutes
Cooking Time: 40 minutes
Servings: 4
Ingredients:
1 ½ tablespoons coconut flour
¼ teaspoon baking powder
1/8 teaspoon salt
1 tablespoon coconut oil, melted
1 whole egg
Directions:
Preheat your oven to 350 °F
Add coconut flour, baking powder, salt
Add coconut oil, eggs and stir well until mixed
Leave the batter for several minutes
Pour half the batter onto the baking pan
Spread it to form a circle, repeat with remaining batter
Bake in the oven for 10 minutes
Once a golden brown texture comes, let it cool and serve
Enjoy!
Nutrition:
Calories: 297
Fat: 14g
Carbohydrates: 15g
Protein: 15g

Chocolate Parfait

Preparation Time: 2 hours
Cooking Time: 0 minutes
Servings: 4
Ingredients:
2 tablespoons cocoa powder

1 cup almond milk

1 tablespoon chia seeds

Pinch of salt

½ teaspoon vanilla extract

Directions:
Take a bowl and add cocoa powder, almond milk, chia seeds, vanilla extract, and stir

Transfer to dessert glass and place in your fridge for 2 hours

Serve and enjoy!

Nutrition:
Calories: 130

Fat: 5g

Carbohydrates: 7g

Protein: 16g

Cauliflower Bagel

Preparation Time: 10 minutes
Cooking Time: 30 minutes
Servings: 12
Ingredients:
1 large cauliflower, divided into florets and roughly chopped
¼ cup nutritional yeast
¼ cup almond flour
½ teaspoon garlic powder
1 ½ teaspoon fine sea salt
2 whole eggs
1 tablespoon sesame seeds

Directions:
Preheat your oven to 400 °F
Line a baking sheet with parchment paper, keep it on the side
Blend cauliflower in a food processor and transfer to a bowl
Add nutritional yeast, almond flour, garlic powder and salt to a bowl, mix
Take another bowl and whisk in eggs, add to cauliflower mix
Give the dough a stir
Incorporate the mix into the egg mix
Make balls from the dough, making a hole using your thumb into each ball
Arrange them on your prepped sheet, flattening them into bagel shapes
Sprinkle sesame seeds and bake for half an hour
Remove the oven and let them cool, enjoy!

Nutrition:
Calories: 152
Fat: 10g
Carbohydrates: 4g
Protein: 4g

Almond Crackers

Preparation Time: 10 minutes
Cooking Time: 20 minutes
Servings: 40 crackers
Ingredients:

1 cup almond flour

¼ teaspoon baking soda

¼ teaspoon salt

1/8 teaspoon black pepper

3 tablespoons sesame seeds

1 egg, beaten

Salt and pepper to taste

Directions:

Preheat your oven to 350 °F

Line two baking sheets with parchment paper and keep them on the side

Mix the dry ingredients into a large bowl and add egg, mix well and form a dough

Divide dough into two balls

Roll out the dough between two pieces of parchment paper

Cut into crackers and transfer them to prep a baking sheet

Bake for 15-20 minutes

Repeat until all the dough has been used up

Leave crackers to cool and serve

Enjoy!

Nutrition:

Calories: 302

Fat: 28g

Carbohydrates: 4g

Protein: 9g

Cashew and Almond Butter

Preparation Time: 5 minutes
Cooking Time: 0 minutes
Servings: 1 ½ cups
Ingredients:
1 cup almonds, blanched
1/3 cup cashew nuts
2 tablespoons coconut oil
Salt as needed
½ teaspoon cinnamon
Directions:
Preheat your oven to 350 °F
Bake almonds and cashews for 12 minutes
Let them cool
Transfer to a food processor and add remaining ingredients
Add oil and keep blending until smooth
Serve and enjoy!
Nutrition:
Calories: 205
Fat: 19g
Carbohydrates: g
Protein: 2.8g

Nut and Chia Mix

Preparation Time: 10 minutes
Cooking Time: 0 minutes
Servings: 1
Ingredients:
1 tablespoon chia seeds
2 cups of water
1 ounce Macadamia nuts
1-2 packets Stevia, optional
1-ounce hazelnuts
Directions:
Add all the listed ingredients to a blender.
Blend on high until smooth and creamy.
Enjoy your smoothie.
Nutrition:
Calories: 452
Fat: 43g
Carbohydrates: 15g
Protein: 9g

Hearty Cucumber Bites

Preparation Time: 5 minutes
Cooking Time: 0 minutes
Servings: 4
Ingredients:
1 (8 ounces) cream cheese container, low fat
1 tablespoon bell pepper, diced
1 tablespoon shallots, diced
1 tablespoon parsley, chopped
2 cucumbers
Pepper to taste
Directions:
Take a bowl and add cream cheese, onion, pepper, parsley
Peel cucumbers and cut in half
Remove seeds and stuff with the cheese mix
Cut into bite-sized portions and enjoy!
Nutrition:
Calories: 85
Fat: 4g
Carbohydrates: 2g
Protein: 3g

Pop Corn Bites

Preparation Time: 5 minutes + 20 minutes chill time
Cooking Time: 2-3 minutes
Servings: 4
Ingredients:
3 cups Medjool dates, chopped
12 ounces brewed coffee
1 cup pecan, chopped
½ cup coconut, shredded
½ cup of cocoa powder

Directions:

Soak dates in warm coffee for 5 minutes

Remove dates from coffee and mash them, making a fine smooth mixture

Stir in remaining ingredients (except cocoa powder) and form small balls out of the mixture

Coat with cocoa powder, serve and enjoy!

Nutrition:

Calories: 265

Fat: 12g

Carbohydrates: 43g

Protein 3g

Hearty Almond Bread

Preparation Time: 15 minutes
Cooking Time: 60 minutes
Servings: 8
Ingredients:

3 cups almond flour

1 teaspoon baking soda

2 teaspoons baking powder

¼ teaspoon sunflower seeds

¼ cup almond milk

½ cup + 2 tablespoons olive oil

3 whole eggs

Directions:

Preheat your oven to 300 ° F

Take a 9x5 inch loaf pan and grease, keep it on the side

Add the listed ingredients to a bowl and pour the batter into the loaf pan

Bake for 60 minutes

Once baked, remove from oven and let it cool

Slice and serve!

Nutrition:

Calories: 277

Fat: 21g

Carbohydrates: 7g

Protein: 10g

Medjool Balls

Preparation Time: 5 minutes + 20 minutes chill time
Cooking Time: 2-3 minutes
Servings: 4
Ingredients:
3 cups Medjool dates, chopped

12 ounces brewed coffee

1 cup pecan, chopped

½ cup coconut, shredded

½ cup of cocoa powder

Directions:
Soak dates in warm coffee for 5 minutes

Remove dates from coffee and mash them, making a fine smooth mixture

Stir in remaining ingredients (except cocoa powder) and form small balls out of the mixture

Coat with cocoa powder, serve and enjoy!

Nutrition:
Calories: 265

Fat: 12g

Carbohydrates: 43g

Protein 3g

Blueberry Pudding

Preparation Time: 20 minutes
Cooking Time: 0 minutes
Servings: 4
Ingredients:
2 cups of frozen blueberries
2 teaspoon of lime zest, grated freshly
20 drops of liquid stevia
½ teaspoon of fresh ginger, grated freshly
4 tablespoon of fresh lime juice
10 tablespoon of water

Directions:
Add all of the listed ingredients to a blender (except blueberries) and pulse the mixture well
Transfer the mix into small serving bowls and chill the bowls
Serve with a topping of blueberries
Enjoy!

Nutrition:
Calories: 166
Fat: 13g
Carbohydrates: 13g
Protein: 1.7g

Chia Seed Pumpkin Pudding

Preparation Time: 10-15 minutes
Cooking Time: 0 minutes
Servings: 4
Ingredients:
1 cup maple syrup
2 teaspoons pumpkin spice
1 cup pumpkin puree
1 ¼ cup of almond milk
½ cup chia seeds

Directions:
Add all of the ingredients to a bowl and gently stir

Let it refrigerate overnight or for at least 15 minutes

Top with your desired ingredients such as blueberries, almonds, etc.

Serve and enjoy!

Nutrition:
Calories: 230
Fat: 10g
Carbohydrates: 22g
Protein: 11g

Parsley Souffle

Preparation Time: 5 minutes
Cooking Time: 6 minutes
Servings: 5
Ingredients:
2 whole eggs
1 fresh red chili pepper, chopped
2 tablespoons coconut cream
1 tablespoon fresh parsley, chopped
Sunflower seeds to taste
Directions:
Preheat your oven to 390 °F
Almond butter two soufflé dishes
Add the ingredients to a blender and mix well
Divide batter into soufflé dishes and bake for 6 minutes
Serve and enjoy!
Nutrition:
Calories: 108
Fat: 9g
Carbohydrates: 9g
Protein: 6g

Mug Cake Popper

Preparation Time: 5 minutes
Cooking Time: 5 minutes
Servings: 2
Ingredients:

2 tablespoons almond flour

1 tablespoon flaxseed meal

1 tablespoon almond butter

1 tablespoon cream cheese

1 large egg

1 bacon, cooked and sliced

½ jalapeno pepper

½ teaspoon baking powder

¼ teaspoon sunflower seeds

Directions:

Take a frying pan and place it over medium heat

Add sliced bacon and cook until they have a crispy texture

Take a microwave proof container and mix all of the listed ingredients (including cooked bacon), clean the sides

Microwave for 75 seconds making sure to put your microwave to high power

Take out the cup and slam it against a surface to take the cake out

Garnish with a bit of jalapeno and serve!

Nutrition:

Calories: 429

Fat: 38g

Carbohydrates: 6g

Protein: 16g

Cinnamon Rice Pudding

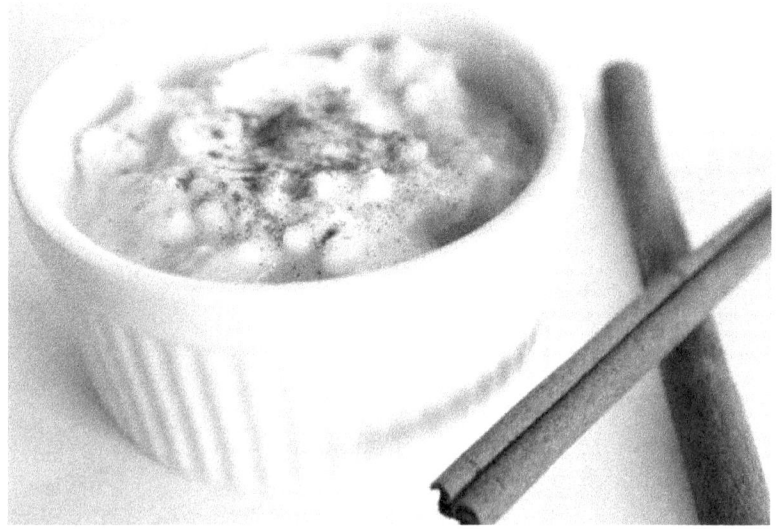

Preparation Time: 10 minutes
Cooking Time: 5 hours
Servings: 4
Ingredients:
6 ½ cups of water
1 cup brown sugar
2 cups white rice
2 cinnamon sticks
½ cup macadamia, shredded
Directions:
Add water, rice, sugar, cinnamon, and coconut to your Slow Cooker
Gently stir
Place lid and cook on HIGH for 5 hours
Discard cinnamon
Divide pudding between dessert dishes and enjoy!

Nutrition:
Calories: 173
Fat: 4g
Carbohydrates: 9g
Protein: 4g

Almond Butter Cookies

Preparation Time: 20 minutes
Cooking Time: 15 minutes
Serving: 36
Ingredients:
Cooking spray
3/4 cup all purpose flour
1/2 cup whole wheat pastry flour, or regular whole wheat flour
3/4 tsp. salt
1 tsp. baking soda
1/4 cup unsalted butter, softened
3/4 cup smooth, unsalted almond butter
1/3 cup packed light brown sugar
1/3 cup granulated sugar
1/2 tsp. vanilla extract
1 egg
36 raw whole almonds

Direction:
Set the oven at 375° and start preheating. Using cooking spray, coat two baking sheets. Whisk baking soda, salt and flours together in a large bowl. Beat sugars, almond butter and butter together in another large bowl till fluffy. Put in egg and vanilla; beat properly till well mixed. Slowly mix in the flour mixture, blending properly.

Form the dough into 3/4-in. balls; arrange on the prepared baking sheets. In the center of each cookie, place an almond and press down slightly. Bake till lightly browned, 10-12 minutes. Remove to a wire rack to cool.

Nutrition:
Calories: 82 calories
Total Carbohydrate: 8.2 g
Cholesterol: 9 mg
Total Fat: 5.1 g
Protein: 1.7 g
Sodium: 87 mg

Conclusion

While you previously likely had very little knowledge about how your kidneys function, their ability to manage mineral and fluid levels in your body, how they synthesize vitamin D so that it's usable by for your cells, and, of course, how they produce Furine through the process of removing toxins and waste from your blood. These organs might be little, but they are mighty. Sadly, over thirty million Americans mighty kidneys are being affected and degraded by chronic kidney disease, high blood pressure, and diabetes.

Thankfully, with the help of Dr. Robert Porter and Dr. Elizabeth Torres, you now have all the information you need to get well on your way to successfully treat your kidney disease! Through a healthy lifestyle and the kidney disease diet, you can halt the damage to your kidneys in its tracks, hopefully preventing the need for dialysis or transplantation in the future. Not only that, but you also learned about some amazing therapies that are now available and will be available in the future, which should give you hope.

If you found the knowledge and information imparted by Dr. Porter and the delicious and nutritious recipes shared by Dr. Torres helpful.

Thank you for reading the Healthy Kidney Cookbook. We hope that with the information you have learned, you will soon gain a healthier and happier lifestyle. You can enjoy gaining healthier kidneys, lower blood pressure, reduced cholesterol, and healthier blood sugar. By combining this with a close relationship with your doctor, you can live better and longer.

www.ingramcontent.com/pod-product-compliance
Lightning Source LLC
Chambersburg PA
CBHW071354210526
45465CB00001B/90